Advance in Orthopedic Trauma Surgery

Advance in Orthopedic Trauma Surgery

Editors

**Steffen Rosslenbroich
Chang-Wug Oh**

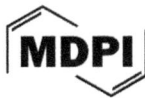

Basel • Beijing • Wuhan • Barcelona • Belgrade • Novi Sad • Cluj • Manchester

Editors
Steffen Rosslenbroich
University Hospital of Muenster
Muenster, Germany

Chang-Wug Oh
Kyungpook National University Hospital
Daegu, Republic of Korea

Editorial Office
MDPI
St. Alban-Anlage 66
4052 Basel, Switzerland

This is a reprint of articles from the Special Issue published online in the open access journal *Journal of Clinical Medicine* (ISSN 2077-0383) (available at: https://www.mdpi.com/journal/jcm/special_issues/Advance_Orthopedic_Trauma_Surgery).

For citation purposes, cite each article independently as indicated on the article page online and as indicated below:

Lastname, A.A.; Lastname, B.B. Article Title. *Journal Name* **Year**, *Volume Number*, Page Range.

ISBN 978-3-0365-9176-6 (Hbk)
ISBN 978-3-0365-9177-3 (PDF)
doi.org/10.3390/books978-3-0365-9177-3

© 2023 by the authors. Articles in this book are Open Access and distributed under the Creative Commons Attribution (CC BY) license. The book as a whole is distributed by MDPI under the terms and conditions of the Creative Commons Attribution-NonCommercial-NoDerivs (CC BY-NC-ND) license.

Contents

Marye M. Méndez-Ojeda, Alejandro Herrera-Rodríguez, Nuria Álvarez-Benito, Himar González-Pacheco, Miguel A. García-Bello, Javier Álvarez-de la Cruz and José L. Pais-Brito
Treatment of Trochanteric Hip Fractures with Cephalomedullary Nails: Single Head Screw vs. Dual Integrated Compression Screw Systems
Reprinted from: *J. Clin. Med.* 2023, 12, 3411, doi:10.3390/jcm12103411 1

Rebecca Sell, Magalie Meinert, Eva Herrmann, Yves Gramlich, Alexander Klug, Oliver Neun, et al.
Preservation of the Subtalar Joint Determines Outcomes in a 10-Year Evaluation of Ankle Arthrodesis
Reprinted from: *J. Clin. Med.* 2023, 12, 3123, doi:10.3390/jcm12093123 13

Harm Hoekstra, Olivier Vinckier, Filip Staes, Lisa Berckmans, Jolien Coninx, Giovanni Matricali, et al.
In Vivo Foot Segmental Motion and Coupling Analysis during Midterm Follow-Up after the Open Reduction Internal Fixation of Trimalleolar Fractures
Reprinted from: *J. Clin. Med.* 2023, 12, 2772, doi:10.3390/jcm12082772 23

Joon-Woo Kim, Chang-Wug Oh, Kyeong-Hyeon Park, Won-Ki Hong, Sung-Hyuk Yoon, Gwang-Sub Lee and Jong-Keon Oh
Application of an Intraoperative Limb Positioner for Adjustable Traction in Both-Column Fractures of the Acetabulum: A Technical Note with Clinical Outcome
Reprinted from: *J. Clin. Med.* 2023, 12, 1682, doi:10.3390/jcm12041682 35

Chang-Wug Oh, Kyeong-Hyeon Park, Joon-Woo Kim, Dong-Hyun Kim, Il Seo, Jin-Han Lee, et al.
Minimally Invasive Derotational Osteotomy of Long Bones: Smartphone Application Used to Improve the Accuracy of Correction
Reprinted from: *J. Clin. Med.* 2023, 12, 1335, doi:10.3390/jcm12041335 43

Claudio Legnani, Matteo Del Re, Marco Viganò, Giuseppe M. Peretti, Enrico Borgo and Alberto Ventura
Relationships between Jumping Performance and Psychological Readiness to Return to Sport 6 Months Following Anterior Cruciate Ligament Reconstruction: A Cross-Sectional Study
Reprinted from: *J. Clin. Med.* 2023, 12, 626, doi:10.3390/jcm12020626 55

Kyeong-Hyeon Park, Chang-Wug Oh, Joon-Woo Kim, Hee-Jun Kim, Dong-Hyun Kim, Jin-Han Lee, et al.
Prophylactic Femoral Neck Fixation in an Osteoporosis Femur Model: A Novel Surgical Technique with Biomechanical Study
Reprinted from: *J. Clin. Med.* 2023, 12, 383, doi:10.3390/jcm12010383 65

Dong-Yang Li, Dong-Xing Lu, Ting Yan, Kai-Yuan Zhang, Bin-Fei Zhang and Yu-Min Zhang
The Association between the Hematocrit at Admission and Preoperative Deep Venous Thrombosis in Hip Fractures in Older People: A Retrospective Analysis
Reprinted from: *J. Clin. Med.* 2023, 12, 353, doi:10.3390/jcm12010353 73

Po-Han Su, Yi-Hsun Huang, Chen-Wei Yeh, Chun-Yen Chen, Yuan-Shun Lo, Hsien-Te Chen and Chun-Hao Tsai
What Are the Key Factors of Functional Outcomes in Patients with Spinopelvic Dissociation Treated with Triangular Osteosynthesis?
Reprinted from: *J. Clin. Med.* 2022, 11, 6715, doi:10.3390/jcm11226715 85

Beom-Soo Kim, Chul-Hyun Cho, Kyung-Jae Lee, Si-Wook Lee and Seok-Ho Byun
Pathomechanism of Triangular Fibrocartilage Complex Injuries in Patients with Distal-Radius Fractures: A Magnetic-Resonance Imaging Study
Reprinted from: *J. Clin. Med.* **2022**, *11*, 6168, doi:10.3390/jcm11206168 . . . . **97**

Xing Wang, Xiang-Dong Wu, Yanbin Zhang, Zhenglin Zhu, Jile Jiang, Guanqing Li, et al.
The Necessity of Implant Removal after Fixation of Thoracolumbar Burst Fractures—A Systematic Review
Reprinted from: *J. Clin. Med.* **2023**, *12*, 2213, doi:10.3390/jcm12062213 . . . . **105**

Pietro Regazzoni, Wen-Chih Liu, Jesse B. Jupiter and Alberto A. Fernandez dell'Oca
Complete Intra-Operative Image Data Including 3D X-rays: A New Format for Surgical Papers Needed?
Reprinted from: *J. Clin. Med.* **2022**, *11*, 7039, doi:10.3390/jcm11237039 . . . . **123**

Antonio Ríos Luna, Homid Fahandezh-Saddi Díaz, Manuel Villanueva Martínez, Ángel Bueno Horcajadas, Roberto Prado, Eduardo Anitua and Sabino Padilla
Reconstruction of Chronic Proximal Hamstring Tear: A Novel Surgical Technique with Semitendinosus Tendon Allograft Assisted with Autologous Plasma Rich in Growth Factors (PRGF)
Reprinted from: *J. Clin. Med.* **2022**, *11*, 5443, doi:10.3390/jcm11185443 . . . . **127**

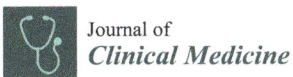

Article

Treatment of Trochanteric Hip Fractures with Cephalomedullary Nails: Single Head Screw vs. Dual Integrated Compression Screw Systems

Marye M. Méndez-Ojeda [1,2], Alejandro Herrera-Rodríguez [1], Nuria Álvarez-Benito [1], Himar González-Pacheco [3], Miguel A. García-Bello [3,4], Javier Álvarez-de la Cruz [1,*] and José L. Pais-Brito [1,2]

1 Orthopedic Surgery and Traumatology Service, University Hospital of the Canary Islands, 38320 La Laguna, Spain; maryemerce@gmail.com (M.M.M.-O.)
2 Orthopaedic Surgery, Health Sciences, Medicine, La Laguna University, 38320 La Laguna, Spain
3 Canary Islands Health Research Institute Foundation (FIISC), 38109 Tenerife, Spain
4 Network for Research on Chronicity, Primary Care, and Health Promotion, (RICAPPS), Spain
* Correspondence: javieralvar.cruz@gmail.com

Abstract: Extracapsular hip fractures are very common in the elderly. They are mainly treated surgically with an intramedullary nail. Nowadays, both endomedullary hip nails with single cephalic screw systems and interlocking double screw systems are available on the market. The latter are supposed to increase rotational stability and therefore decrease the risk of collapse and cut-out. A retrospective cohort study was carried out, in which 387 patients with extracapsular hip fracture undergoing internal fixation with an intramedullary nail were included to study the occurrence of complications and reoperations. Of the 387 patients, 69% received a single head screw nail and 31% received a dual integrated compression screw nail. The median follow-up was 1.1 years, and in that time, a total of 17 reoperations were performed (4.2%; 2.1% for single head screw nails vs. 8.7% for double head screws). According to the multivariate logistic regression model adjusted for age, sex and basicervical fracture, the adjusted hazard risk of reoperation required was 3.6 times greater when using double interlocking screw systems ($p = 0.017$). A propensity scores analysis confirmed this finding. In conclusion, despite the potential benefits of using two interlocking head screw systems and the increased risk of reoperation in our single center, we encourage to other researchers to explore this question in a wider multicenter study.

Keywords: hip fracture; trochanteric fracture; Gamma nail; InterTAN nail

1. Introduction

Hip fractures (HF) are a frequent problem in elderly patients, and are related to osteopenia and osteoporosis. Around 1.6 million patients suffer from HF per year [1], and by 2050, the global incidence is believed to become 4.5 million [2]. Reduced bone density, female sex (female/male ratio greater than 2/1 in those over 50 years of age), low weight and reduced physical activity are main risk factors for HF [1,2]. The mortality rate among patients who suffer a hip fracture is 5–10% one month after the fracture and 20–30% in the first year [1,2].

Hip fractures can be classified as intracapsular or extracapsular, and the latter are subdivided into basicervical, intertrochanteric/pertrochanteric and subtrochanteric. Up to half of such fractures are intertrochanteric, usually occurring in elderly patients as a result of low-energy trauma [3]. The main treatment of these trochanteric fractures is surgery, which can be extramedullary or intramedullary. Previously, extramedullary treatment with sliding hip screw (SHS) was the most indicated, but some studies showed that nailing gave better fracture fixation results for uncommon trochanteric fractures, especially subtrochanteric fractures, so the use of nailing has dramatically increased even though there is no evidence that it is superior to the SHS in a simple intertrochanteric pattern [3].

Some of the most-used intramedullary nailing alternatives in our region are the Gamma3 nail, PFNA (Proximal Femoral Nail Antirotation) and TRIGEN InterTAN. The latter differs from the others in that it offers the possibility of two cephalo-cervical screws that provide linear compression and additional resistance to the rotation of the femoral head, while the others use a single screw [4,5]. Several studies and meta-analyses have compared the use of these methods of treatment without reaching a definitive conclusion on which fixation method is most appropriate to reduce complications and improve prognosis [6–17]. Independent risk factors for early mortality already reported in the literature are: male sex, dependence on others for the basic activities of daily living, American Society of Anesthesiologists (ASA) score > 2, older age and medical complications occurring while an inpatient [18]. Fracture stability also plays a key role in the prognosis for these patients, not only influencing early device failure requiring reoperation within 12 months, but also increasing the rate of mortality after trochanteric hip fractures by up to 1.6 times [19]. Studies such as Chehade et al. also describe an increase in early osteosynthesis failure associated with the use of double lag screw systems [19]. Attending to only unstable hip fractures, such as subtrochanteric fractures, Panteli et al. identified six risk factors associated with reoperation: age < 75 years old, pre-injury femoral neck shaft angle, choice of nail, varus reduction angle, fracture-related infection and non-union. The addition of a proximal anti-rotation screw did not confer any benefit [20] in terms of reoperation or survival rates. Figures 1 and 2 show typical cases of pertrochanteric hip fracture treated with an endomedullary nail.

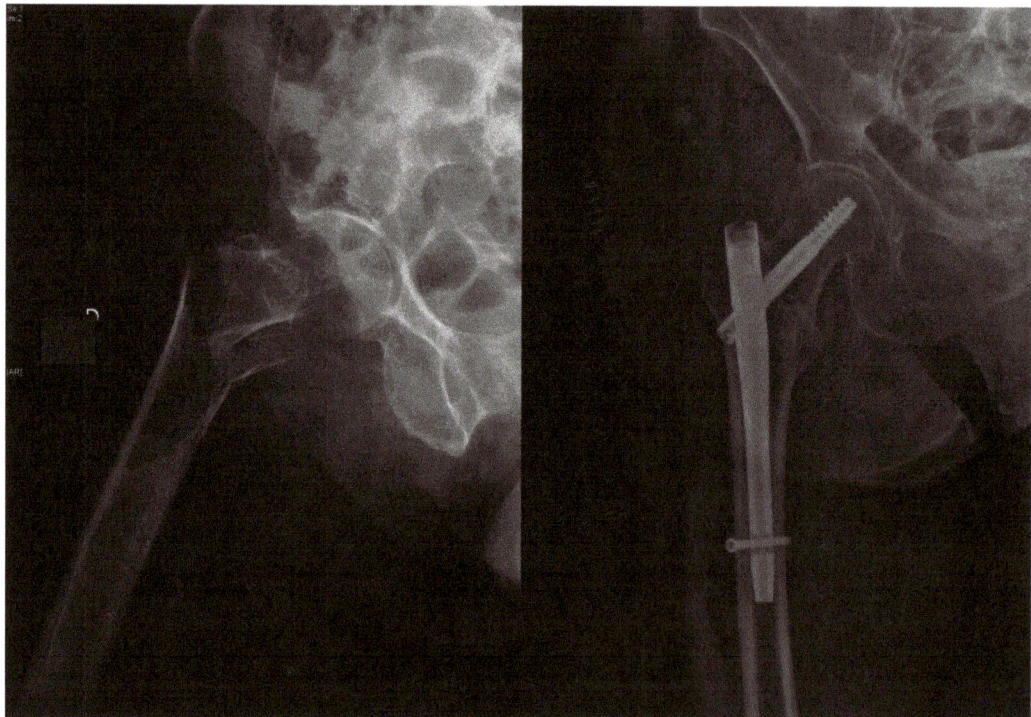

Figure 1. Pertrocantheric hip fracture treated with a short Gamma3 nail.

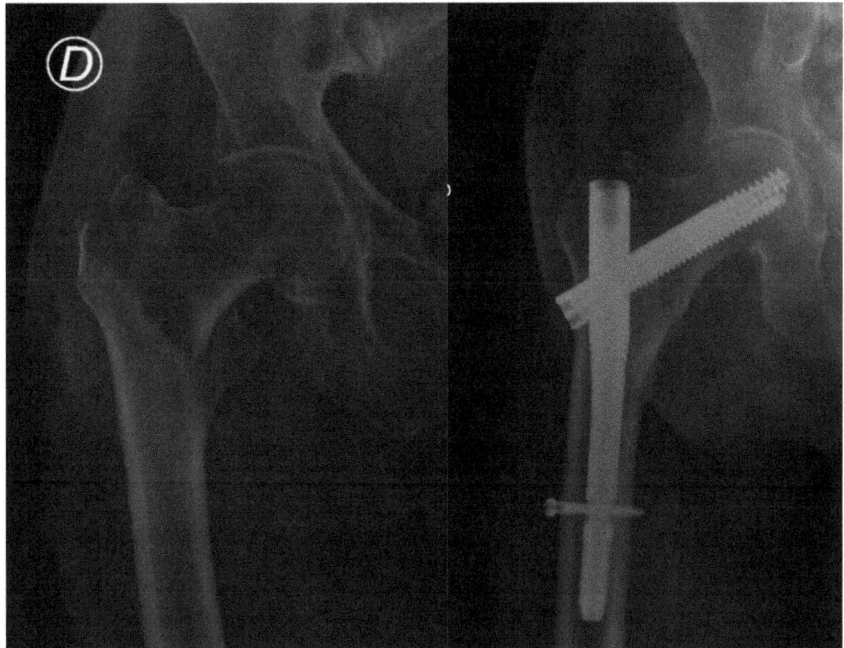

Figure 2. Pertrocantheric hip fracture treated with a short InterTAN nail (letter D for right lower limb).

For a time, in our service, we had the impression that systems with two cephalo-cervical screws had a higher rate of reoperations. As such, the aim of this study is to retrospectively review major post-surgical complications as they relate to the type of nail used, comparing single head screw nails to dual integrated compression screw nails, with nails being implanted at a third-level hospital. The hypothesis of our study is that cephalomedullary nailing with double head screw systems present a greater number of post-surgical complications compared to single screw systems.

2. Materials and Methods

2.1. Study Design

Single-center retrospective cohort study.

2.2. Study Subjects

We collected data of patients who underwent surgery and received a single or double head screw hip nail at the Hospital Universitario de Canarias between 1 April 2019 and 26 July 2021 Inclusion Criteria: patients who received a single or double head screw intramedullary hip nail, both short and long. All patients included began rehabilitation treatment with full weight-bearing authorized in the first 24 h after the procedure, as long as the postoperative hemoglobin level was greater than 8 g/dL in the postoperative analysis. Exclusion Criteria: absence of follow-up, use of another fixation system other than the Gamma3 or TRIGEN InterTAN nail, shaft femoral fractures, patients who underwent surgery more than 72 h after suffering the fracture.

In our service, all pertrochanteric, basicervical or subtrochanteric fractures are treated with endomedullary hip nails. Both Gamma3 and InterTAN nails are available in stock, and the choice of implant is at the discretion of the attending physician. Both short and long nails were included. Short nails have been selected for stable fracture patterns (AO/OTA classification 31.A2/31.A3) and long nails for unstable fracture patterns (31.A3).

Fracture patterns classified as 31.A2 were treated at the surgeon's discretion according to his clinical judgment.

2.3. Study Variables

Age, sex (female/male), laterality (right/left), type of fracture (AO classification), date of surgery, type of nail (Gamma3/TRIGEN InterTAN), reoperation (yes/no; considering only the first reoperation and the time until first reoperation), reason for reoperation (cut-out/implant failure/infection/others), date of reoperation, exitus and date of exitus.

2.4. Data Collection

After approval by the Ethics Committee of the Hospital Universitario de Canarias (code CHUC_2021_134), all patients who met the inclusion criteria and none of the exclusion criteria were identified. A Microsoft Excel-type document was prepared in which patient data related to all study variables were collected, excluding patients' personal data. All patient medical records were reviewed through the computer system of University Hospital of the Canary Islands to complete the document, and the following data were collected: evolution of hospitalization, discharge reports, follow-up in outpatient consultations.

2.5. Statistical Analysis

A descriptive analysis of the sample was made, where the continuous variables were expressed by means and standard deviations (SD), and categorical variables expressed through frequencies and percentages. In addition, a bivariate analysis was carried out using the t-student or chi-square test according to the nature of the variables (continuous or categorical, respectively).

In order to compare post-surgical complications requiring re-intervention, a survival cox regression model was applied. The dependent variable in the model was a dichotomous variable indicating whether reoperation was required (yes/no) and the time until reoperation. The following covariates were included in the model: type of nail (Gamma3/InterTAN), type of fracture (Basicervical/Other), age and sex. Additionally, due to concerns related to the rule of ten outcome events per predictor variable, the effect was also estimated using full propensity score matching with the MatchIt package, which is particularly suitable for modeling rare events.

3. Results

A total of 387 medical records were analyzed. The Gamma3 nail was used in 262 patients (67.7%) and InterTAN was used in 125 patients (32.3%). The mean age of the study population was 81.6 (SD = 11.3), of which 74.2% were women (Table 1). The patients were followed up with for a median of 1.1 years, with a maximum follow-up of 2.6 years.

Table 1. Characteristics of the sample according to the type of nail.

	Total (n = 387)	Gamma3 (n = 262)	InterTAN (n = 125)	p-Value
Age, mean (SD)	81.6 (11.3)	81.9 (10.7)	81.1 (12.5)	0.524
Gender, Female, n (%)	287 (74.2%)	191 (72.9%)	96 (76.8%)	0.487
Laterality, right side, n (%)	213 (55.0%)	140 (53.4%)	73 (58.4%)	0.419
Type of fracture, n (%)				<0.001
Intertrochanteric	240 (62%)	170 (64.9%)	70 (56%)	0.116
Persubtrochanteric	52 (13.4%)	36 (13.7%)	16 (12.8%)	0.925
Basicervical	51 (13.2%)	19 (7.3%)	32 (25.6%)	<0.001
Subtrochanteric	44 (11.4%)	37 (14.1%)	7 (5.6%)	0.022

SD = Standard Deviation.

A comparison of the sample based on the type of nail revealed that the two groups had similar characteristics, with no significant differences in age, sex, laterality, or mortality. However, there were some variations in the type of fracture observed. In the InterTAN group, 25.6% of the fractures were basicervical, while 7.3% of the Gamma3 nail group had basicervical fractures ($p < 0.001$). Conversely, the Gamma3 nail group had a higher percentage of subtrochanteric fractures (14.1%) compared to the InterTAN group (5.6%; $p = 0.022$). There was no significant difference in the percentage of intertrochanteric fractures between the two groups ($p = 0.116$) (Table 1).

A total of 17 fractures required reoperation, as shown in Table 2. The reoperation rates were higher in InterTAN group compared to the Gamma3 group ($p = 0.009$). Analysis indicates that cut-out may have been a contributing factor to the difference in reoperation rates between the two groups ($p = 0.016$).

Table 2. Incidence of complications in the follow-up period after surgery.

	Total (n = 387)	Gamma3 (n = 262)	InterTAN (n = 125)	p-Value
Median of follow up (P25–P75)	1.1 (0.5–1.8)	1.0 (0.5–1.8)	1.2 (0.6–1.7)	0.82
Reoperations in the follow-up period after surgery, n (%)	17 & (4.4%)	6 (2.3%)	11 & (8.8%)	0.008
Reoperation required, rates at 1.5 Years Following Surgery *, %	5.8%	1.9%	13.3%	0.009
Any complication, rates at 1.5 Years Following Surgery, n (%)	18 (4.7%)	6 (2.3%)	12 (9.6%)	0.003
Cut-out	8 (2.1%)	2 (0.8%)	6 (4.8%)	0.016
Peri-implant fracture	6 (1.6%)	2 (0.8%)	4 (3.2%)	0.089
Nail Tear	3 (0.8%)	1 (0.4%)	2 (1.6%)	0.245
Infection	1 (0.3%)	1 (0.4%)	0	>0.99
Second reoperation in the follow-up period after surgery, n (%)	2 (0.5%)	1 (0.8%)	0	0.54
Exitus Rates at 1.5 Year Following Surgery *, %	26.9%	26.4%	27.8%	0.79

* Kaplan-Meier curve survival estimations. & One InterTAN patient required a reoperation, but it was ruled out due to health problems.

Analyzing which other factor could explain the reoperation rate, we can see there was no significant different rate associated with the side of the fracture ($p = 0.80$), sex ($p = 0.50$) or age ($p = 0.45$).

3.1. Risk of Reoperation in the Follow-Up Adjusting by Cox Regression Modeling

The Cox regression model was used to analyze the association between the risk of reoperation and different covariates. The results of the model indicate that the type of nail (Gamma3/InterTAN) was a significant predictor of reoperation, with patients who received the InterTAN having a higher hazard ratio (HR) of 3.6 (95% CI: 1.3, 10.5) for required reoperation compared to those who received the Gamma3 nail. The results of Model 2 (Cox regression model for risk of reoperation needed) indicate that the type of nail (Gamma3 vs. InterTAN) was a significative predictor of reoperation required (Table 3), but neither the type of fracture (basicervical/other) nor age nor sex were found to be significant predictors. These results suggest that the type of nail may be an important factor in determining the risk of reoperation after surgery.

In addition to the Cox regression analysis, a Kaplan-Meier survival curve was generated to visualize the probability of required reoperation over time for the different nails. The results of the Kaplan-Meier analysis show that the probability of required reoperation was higher for patients who received the InterTAN (Figure 3a). The curve for the InterTAN group drops more steeply than the curve for the Gamma3 nail group, indicating that reoperations required were more likely to occur early on, and at a higher rate in the InterTAN group. We can see that the difference was important from one year of follow-up. Additionally, the log-rank test was performed to test the equality of the survival curves between the two groups, with a $p = 0.001$ indicating a statistically significant difference between the groups. Overall, the Kaplan-Meier analysis provides a visual representation of the reoperation required rates, and supports the findings from the Cox regression analysis. Otherwise, we analyzed all-cause mortality and didn't find any difference between nail groups related to overall survival, $p = 0.70$ (Figure 3b).

Table 3. Cox regression model for risk of reoperation needed.

	Model 1: Not Including Type of Nail		Model 2: Including Type of Nail	
	HR [95% CI]	*p*-Value	HR [95% CI]	*p*-Value
InterTAN vs. Gamma3 nail	-	-	3.6 [1.3–10.5]	0.017
Basicervical fracture	2.3 [0.82–6.7]	0.11	1.4 [0.47–4.3]	0.54
Age	0.99 [0.95–1.03]	0.70	1.0 [0.96–1.04]	0.94
Men	1.3 [0.41–4.1]	0.66	1.4 [0.43–4.4]	0.58
McFadden pseudo-R2	0.017		0.052	

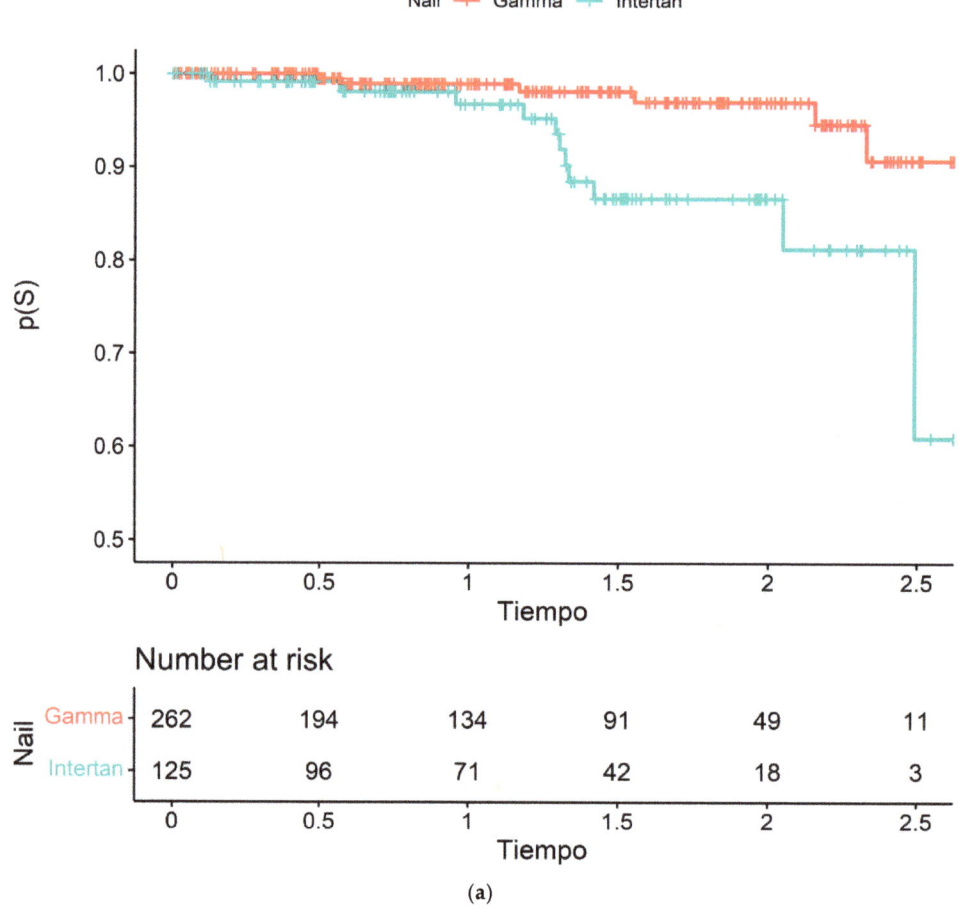

(a)

Figure 3. *Cont.*

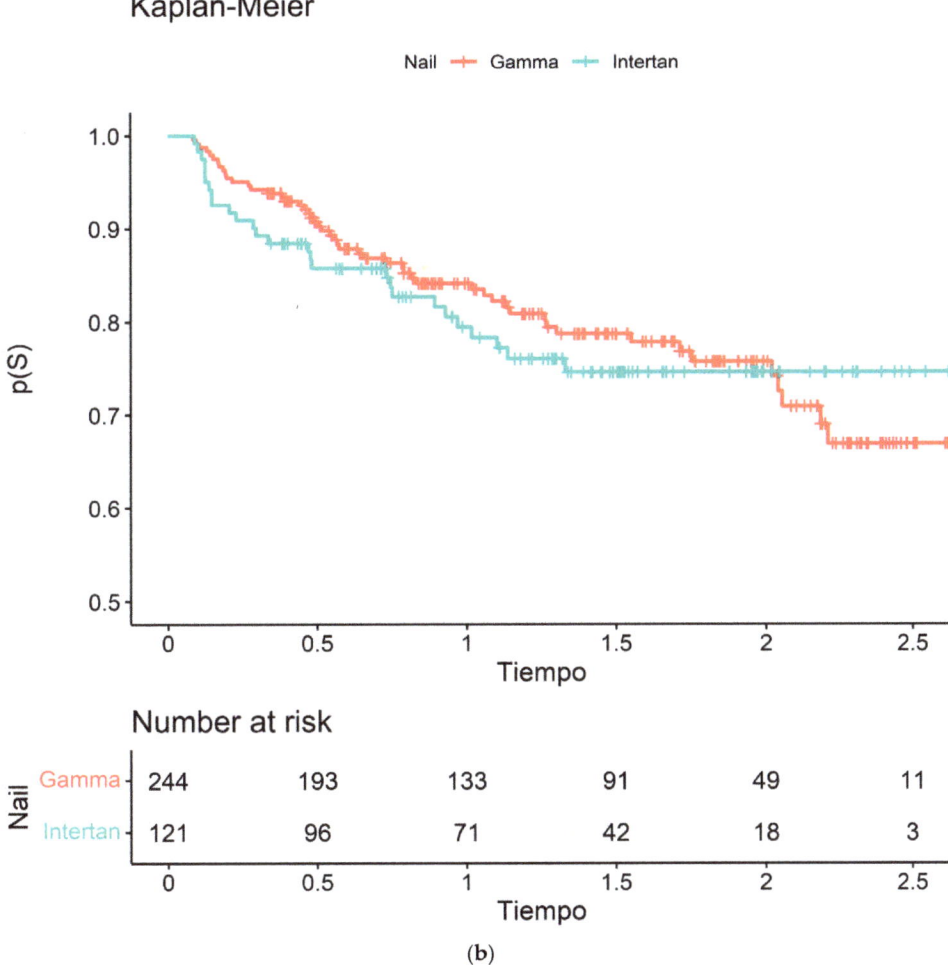

Figure 3. (**a**) Risk of reoperation needed. (**b**) Risk of all-cause mortality.

3.2. Risk of Reoperation Evaluated after Propensity Score Matching

We conducted a propensity score matching, which shows how the balance of the baseline covariates between the treatment groups was assessed to evaluate the success of the matching procedure. The results after propensity score matching show that the distribution of the baseline characteristics, including age, sex and type of fracture, were similar between the treatment groups, with a standardized mean difference of less than 0.1 for all covariates (Figure 4). This suggests that the propensity score matching procedure was successful in controlling for potential confounding effects of the baseline covariates on the treatment effect. Additionally, the effect of the treatment on the outcome of interest, reoperation, was found to be consistent with the results obtained before propensity score matching (HR = 3.3; $p = 0.038$).

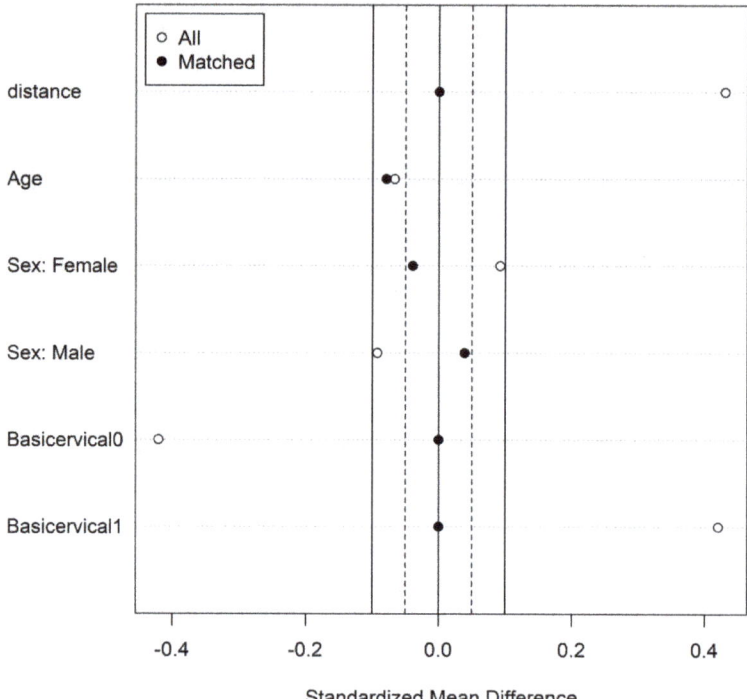

Figure 4. Standardized mean difference of baseline characteristics before and after propensity score matching. The solid vertical line represents the threshold of 0.1, indicating balance between the groups. The matching procedure was successful in balancing the baseline characteristics between the treatment groups.

4. Discussion

The present study showed that in this cohort, double interlocking head screw nailing systems such as the InterTAN nail led to a significantly higher rate of reoperations compared to the Gamma3 nail. At first, it seemed that this finding could be associated with the fracture pattern, as there was a heterogenous distribution of types of fracture. However, no significant differences were found in any other indicators between the two groups, including type of fracture, sex or age.

Although there is some scientific biomechanical proof of the rotational stability of InterTAN nails [5], in clinical studies and reviews, there is still controversy between the existing types of nails [6–17]. A priori, this increase in rotational stability would be advantageous in basicervical fracture traces by avoiding rotation of the cervical neck when drilling or inserting the cephalic screw. However, this supposed biomechanical advantage was not reflected in the patients in the study who underwent surgery.

There have been two Cochrane reviews about trochanteric fracture treatment [3,7]. One compares nails to extramedullary implants [4] and another compares the different types of nails [8]. In the latter review, Queally et al. analyzed 17 randomized clinical trials (RCTs) prior to 2014, compared different nails and concluded that there was insufficient evidence from randomized trials to determine if there are important differences in patient outcomes between the different designs of proximal femoral intramedullary nail produced by different manufacturers when used for the fixation of unstable, or stable, trochanteric fractures [7].

There are also more recent clinical trials and meta-analyses comparing different nails and it continues to be uncertain whether there is a difference between implants. Two RCTs specifically compared Gamma3 to InterTAN with similar results [8,9]. Su et al. concluded that no significant difference was found in X-ray times, reduction results, TAD, time to mobilization, operative complications, femoral neck shortening or fracture healing time [8]. Berger et al. affirmed that, in terms of implant-related complications, no significant differences were recorded [9]. Zhang et al. have several studies, including one RCT, comparing InterTAN to PFNA-II in which they didn't find any significant differences in outcomes except for high pain [10–12]. Ülkü et al. retrospectively studied nail migration. Although there was a significant difference in favor of InterTAN, nail migration in the PFNA group did not result in reoperation [13]. Ricci et al. also found a higher radiological collapse in PFNA and DHS vs. InterTAN, but they don't mention whether that has clinical repercussions [14]. The Liu et al. meta-analysis included two RCTs and seven observational studies, and concluded that patients with the InterTAN nail had a lower risk of screw migration, pain at thigh or hip, cutout, varus collapse of the femoral head, femoral shaft fracture and reoperation. Nonetheless, that finding was based mainly on observational studies, as the researchers didn't find superiority in cutout, reoperation and femoral shaft fracture when considering only the RCTs [15]. There are two other meta-analyses that suggest that InterTAN leads to fewer complications when compared to single screw devices. However, both of them include mainly retrospective studies and both have conflicts of interest, as they were done by Smith and Nephew collaborators [16,17].

Although we have not screened every patient included in the study for osteoporosis, we can affirm that most patients suffered from it to a greater or lesser degree due to their age, comorbidities and the fact that they had suffered the fracture from a low energy impact. A plausible explanation for these results could be the greater aggression to both the head and the femoral neck caused by the integrated double screw. The double reaming performed, coupled with the fact that the double screw system is thicker than the single screw, could further weaken the cortices and the vascularization of an already-weakened bone, increasing the risk of osteosynthesis failure in certain cases.

However, there are several inherent limitations to our study that deserve consideration. First, the retrospective nature presents a potential selection bias. Patients were distributed between treatment groups based on surgeon preference and we didn't consider the surgeon's experience in our analysis. Additionally, the pattern of fracture was heterogeneously distributed in both groups and the number of cases is low. Although adjustment was made for several variables, it is possible that residual confounders between the nails could still be present, and therefore the adjusted cox regression and propensity score matching may not be able to adjust or balance all unmeasured confounders. In our center, immediate postoperative radiographs are performed by radiology technicians without the direct supervision and approval of a traumatologist. In several patients, the axial projection of the hip was not performed correctly or was not performed at all. Due of this, it was not possible to perform a correct measurement of the tip-apex distance in all patients, so it was decided not to include it in the study parameters. Lastly, single-center studies lack the external validation required to support changes in practice, so we recommend interpreting these results with caution.

5. Conclusions

Single head screw nails such as Gamma3 and dual integrated compression head screw nails such as InterTAN may be effective for surgical treatment of trochanteric fractures.

A higher risk of reoperation was found when using InterTAN. Therefore, despite the potential biomechanical benefits of using two screws with the InterTAN nail, we cannot recommend it over the Gamma3 nail.

Large-sample multicenter studies may be needed in the future to compare the different cephalomedullary nails available.

Author Contributions: Conceptualization, M.M.M.-O.; methodology M.M.M.-O.; software A.H.-R. and M.A.G.-B.; validation, J.L.P.-B.; formal analysis, A.H.-R., M.A.G.-B. and H.G.-P.; investigation, M.M.M.-O.; resources, M.M.M.-O.; data curation, A.H.-R., M.A.G.-B. and J.Á.-d.l.C.; writing—original draft A.H.-R.; preparation J.Á.-d.l.C. and A.H.-R.; writing—review and editing, N.Á.-B.; visualization, N.Á.-B. and J.Á.-d.l.C.; supervision, J.L.P.-B.; project administration, M.M.M.-O.; funding acquisition, not necessary. All authors have read and agreed to the published version of the manuscript.

Funding: This research received no external funding.

Institutional Review Board Statement: The study was conducted in accordance with the Declaration of Helsinki, and approved by the Institutional Review Board (or Ethics Committee) of University Hospital of the Canary Islands (protocol code CHUC_2021_134; date of approval: 27 January 2022).

Informed Consent Statement: Informed consent was obtained from all subjects involved in the study.

Data Availability Statement: The data presented in this study are openly available in Figshare at https://doi.org/10.6084/m9.figshare.21548340.v2 (accessed on 3 May 2023).

Conflicts of Interest: The authors declare no conflict of interest.

References

1. Huette, P.; Abou-Arab, O.; Djebara, A.-E.; Terrasi, B.; Beyls, C.; Guinot, P.-G.; Havet, E.; Dupont, H.; Lorne, E.; Ntouba, A.; et al. Risk Factors and Mortality of Patients Undergoing Hip Fracture Surgery: A One-Year Follow-up Study. *Sci. Rep.* **2020**, *10*, 9607. [CrossRef] [PubMed]
2. Aubrun, F. Fracture de l'extrémité Supérieure Du Fémur Du Patient Âgé: Aspect Épidémiologique, Facteurs de Risque. *Ann. Fr. Ann. Anesth. Resusc.* **2011**, *30*, e37–e39. [CrossRef] [PubMed]
3. Park, M.J.; Handoll, H.H. Gamma and Other Cephalocondylic Intramedullary Nails versus Extramedullary Implants for Extracapsular Hip Fractures in Adults. *Cochrane Database Syst. Rev.* **2008**, *16*, CD000093. [CrossRef]
4. Date, A.; Panthula, M.; Bolina, A. Comparison of Clinical and Radiological Outcomes in Intertrochanteric Fractures Treated with InterTAN Nail against Conventional Cephalomedullary Nails: A Systematic Review. *Future Sci. OA* **2021**, *7*, FSO668. [CrossRef] [PubMed]
5. Santoni, B.G.; Diaz, M.A.; Stoops, T.K.; Lannon, S.; Ali, A.; Sanders, R.W. Biomechanical Investigation of an Integrated 2-Screw Cephalomedullary Nail Versus a Sliding Hip Screw in Unstable Intertrochanteric Fractures. *J. Orthop. Trauma* **2019**, *33*, 82–87. [CrossRef] [PubMed]
6. Ma, K.-L.; Wang, X.; Luan, F.-J.; Xu, H.-T.; Fang, Y.; Min, J.; Luan, H.-X.; Yang, F.; Zheng, H.; He, S.-J. Proximal Femoral Nails Antirotation, Gamma Nails, and Dynamic Hip Screws for Fixation of Intertrochanteric Fractures of Femur: A Meta-Analysis. *Orthop. Traumatol. Surg. Res.* **2014**, *100*, 859–866. [CrossRef] [PubMed]
7. Queally, J.M.; Harris, E.; Handoll, H.H.; Parker, M.J. Intramedullary Nails for Extracapsular Hip Fractures in Adults. *Cochrane Database Syst. Rev.* **2014**, *9*, CD004961. [CrossRef] [PubMed]
8. Su, H.; Sun, K.; Wang, X. A Randomized Prospective Comparison of InterTAN and Gamma3 for Treating Unstable Intertrochanteric Fractures. *Int. J. Clin. Exp. Med.* **2016**, *9*, 8640–8647.
9. Berger-Groch, J.; Rupprecht, M.; Schoepper, S.; Schroeder, M.; Rueger, J.M.; Hoffmann, M. Five-Year Outcome Analysis of Intertrochanteric Femur Fractures: A Prospective Randomized Trial Comparing a 2-Screw and a Single-Screw Cephalomedullary Nail. *J. Orthop. Trauma* **2016**, *30*, 483–488. [CrossRef] [PubMed]
10. Zhang, S.; Zhang, K.; Jia, Y.; Yu, B.; Feng, W. InterTan Nail Versus Proximal Femoral Nail Antirotation-Asia in the Treatment of Unstable Trochanteric Fractures. *Orthopedics* **2013**, *36*, 182. [CrossRef] [PubMed]
11. Zhang, C.; Xu, B.; Liang, G.; Zeng, X.; Zeng, D.; Chen, D.; Ge, Z.; Yu, W.; Zhang, X. Optimizing Stability in AO/OTA 31-A2 Intertrochanteric Fracture Fixation in Older Patients with Osteoporosis. *J. Int. Med. Res.* **2018**, *46*, 1767–1778. [CrossRef] [PubMed]
12. Zhang, H.; Zhu, X.; Pei, G.; Zeng, X.; Zhang, N.; Xu, P.; Chen, D.; Yu, W.; Zhang, X. A Retrospective Analysis of the InterTan Nail and Proximal Femoral Nail Anti-Rotation in the Treatment of Intertrochanteric Fractures in Elderly Patients with Osteoporosis: A Minimum Follow-up of 3 Years. *J. Orthop. Surg. Res.* **2017**, *12*, 147. [CrossRef] [PubMed]
13. Ülkü, T.K.; Tok, O.; Seyhan, M.; Gereli, A.; Kaya, A. Comparison of Third Generation Proximal Femoral Nails in Treatment of Reverse Oblique Intertrochanteric Fractures. *Bezmialem Sci.* **2019**, *7*, 271–275. [CrossRef]
14. Ricci, M.J.; McAndrew, C.M.; Miller, A.N.; Kamath, G.; Ricci, W.M. Are Two-Part Intertrochanteric Femur Fractures Stable and Does Stability Depend on Fixation Method? *J. Orthop. Trauma* **2019**, *33*, 428–431. [CrossRef] [PubMed]
15. Liu, W.; Liu, J.; Ji, G. Comparison of Clinical Outcomes with Proximal Femoral Nail Anti-Rotation versus InterTAN Nail for Intertrochanteric Femoral Fractures: A Meta-Analysis. *J. Orthop. Surg. Res.* **2020**, *15*, 500. [CrossRef] [PubMed]
16. Nherera, L.; Trueman, P.; Horner, A.; Watson, T.; Johnstone, A.J. Comparison of a Twin Interlocking Derotation and Compression Screw Cephalomedullary Nail (InterTAN) with a Single Screw Derotation Cephalomedullary Nail (Proximal Femoral Nail Antirotation): A Systematic Review and Meta-Analysis for Intertrochanteric Fractures. *J. Orthop. Surg. Res.* **2018**, *13*, 46. [CrossRef] [PubMed]

17. Quartley, M.; Chloros, G.; Papakostidis, K.; Saunders, C.; Giannoudis, P.V. Stabilisation of AO OTA 31-A Unstable Proximal Femoral Fractures: Does the Choice of Intramedullary Nail Affect the Incidence of Post-Operative Complications? A Systematic Literature Review and Meta-Analysis. *Injury* **2022**, *53*, 827–840. [CrossRef] [PubMed]
18. Smith, T.; Pelpola, K.; Ball, M.; Ong, A.; Myint, P.K. Pre-Operative Indicators for Mortality Following Hip Fracture Surgery: A Systematic Review and Meta-Analysis. *Age Ageing* **2014**, *43*, 464–471. [CrossRef] [PubMed]
19. Chehade, M.J.; Carbone, T.; Awwad, D.; Taylor, A.; Wildenauer, C.; Ramasamy, B.; McGee, M. Influence of Fracture Stability on Early Patient Mortality and Reoperation After Pertrochanteric and Intertrochanteric Hip Fractures. *J. Orthop. Trauma.* **2015**, *29*, 538–543. [CrossRef] [PubMed]
20. Panteli, M.; Vun, J.S.H.; West, R.M.; Howard, A.; Pountos, I.; Giannoudis, P.V. Subtrochanteric Femoral Fractures and Intramedullary Nailing Complications: A Comparison of Two Implants. *J. Orthop. Traumatol.* **2022**, *23*, 27. [CrossRef] [PubMed]

Disclaimer/Publisher's Note: The statements, opinions and data contained in all publications are solely those of the individual author(s) and contributor(s) and not of MDPI and/or the editor(s). MDPI and/or the editor(s) disclaim responsibility for any injury to people or property resulting from any ideas, methods, instructions or products referred to in the content.

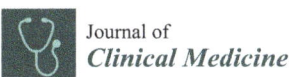

Article

Preservation of the Subtalar Joint Determines Outcomes in a 10-Year Evaluation of Ankle Arthrodesis

Rebecca Sell [1], Magalie Meinert [2], Eva Herrmann [3], Yves Gramlich [2], Alexander Klug [2], Oliver Neun [1], Reinhard Hoffmann [2] and Sebastian Fischer [1,*]

[1] Department of Foot and Ankle Surgery, Berufsgenossenschaftliche Unfallklinik Frankfurt am Main, 60389 Frankfurt am Main, Germany
[2] Department for Trauma and Orthopaedic Surgery, Berufsgenossenschaftliche Unfallklinik Frankfurt am Main, 60389 Frankfurt am Main, Germany
[3] Institut für Biostatistik und Mathematische Modellierung, Goethe-Universität Frankfurt am Main, Theodor-Stern-Kai 7, 60596 Frankfurt am Main, Germany
* Correspondence: sebastian.fischer@bgu-frankfurt.de

Abstract: Posttraumatic osteoarthritis may lead to surgical fusion of the ankle joint if non-surgical therapy fails. The indication for a fusion of the joint is based on the pain and disability of the patient, radiographic imaging, and surgeon experience, with no strict guidelines. We aimed to compare outcomes after tibiotalocalcaneal arthrodesis (TTCA) and tibiotalar arthrodesis (TTA) to highlight the functional importance of the subtalar joint. In total, 432 patients with ankle arthrodesis were retrospectively enrolled. Group A ($n = 216$) underwent TTCA; group B ($n = 216$) underwent TTA. Demographics, Olerud & Molander Ankle Score (OMAS), Foot Function Index (FFI-D), and Short Form-12 Questionnaire (SF-12) were recorded at a mean follow-up of 6.2 years. The mean OMAS was 50.7; the mean FFI-D was 68.9; the mean SF-12 physical component summary was 39.1. These scores differed significantly between the groups ($p < 0.001$). The overall revision rate was 18%, primarily for revision of non-union and infection ($p < 0.001$). Approximately 16% of group A and 26% of group B were able to return to previous work ($p < 0.001$). Based on significantly worse clinical scores of TTCA compared to TTA and the prolonged downtime and permanent incapacity, the indication for a generous subtalar joint arthrodesis with planned ankle arthrodesis should always be critically examined.

Keywords: ankle arthrodesis; tibiotalocalcaneal arthrodesis; subtalar arthrodesis; gait pattern; posttraumatic osteoarthritis

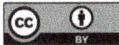

1. Introduction

Rare primary arthroses of the ankle joint account for less than ten percent of all cases. Additionally, traffic accidents and sports injuries lead to serious fractures of the ankle joint with posttraumatic osteoarthritis [1]. However, chronic instabilities due to insufficiency of the inner and outer ligaments of the upper ankle joint, as well as acute and chronic syndesmosis injuries with resultant chronic instability, are also possible causes, and habitual malpositions with an axial deviation of the hindfoot or entire leg axis also favor such signs of wear and tear [2]. If non-surgical therapy, such as adjustment of footwear, nonsteroidal anti-inflammatory drugs, and physiotherapy, fails, and joint preservation is no longer possible, the indication for arthrodesis of the ankle joint arises.

In this context, it is known that a subsequent conversion of a total ankle replacement into a tibiotalar arthrodesis is inferior to a primary fusion [3,4]. The idea that previously mild osteoarthritis of the subtalar joint may develop into severe osteoarthritis leads to a discussion of early indications for tibiotalocalcaneal arthrodesis (TTCA).

Regardless of the radiological findings, complaints of pain surrounding the subtalar joint cannot always be reliably differentiated when tibiotalar arthrodesis (TTA) is indicated.

The indication for TTA or TTCA then depends primarily on the experience of the treating surgeon, in addition to the patient's disability and pain.

The outcomes of TTA and TTCA are sometimes unsatisfactory and are associated with low score values due to the associated restriction of movement and the long duration of pain and suffering [5,6]. We aimed to compare the clinical outcomes of TTCA and TTA in a direct comparison using a demographically comparable and large patient population.

2. Materials and Methods

2.1. Population

Between 2010 and 2022, 432 patients with ankle arthrodesis (278 males and 154 females, mean age: 64 years [range: 27–93 years]) were retrospectively enrolled in this comparative monocentric study. Group A (n = 216) underwent TTCA; group B (n = 216) underwent TTA. Both groups were equally distributed in terms of demographics (Table 1). All patients were seen during foot surgery consultations at the study center (Figure 1). The diagnosis of end-stage posttraumatic osteoarthritis of the ankle was made on the basis of clinical examination, obligatory weight-bearing radiographs, and computer tomography.

Table 1. Patient characteristics.

Characteristic		TTC (n = 216)	TT (n = 216)	All (n = 432)	p
Follow-up (months)	Mean	78.61	69.48	73.99	0.018
	SEM	2.73	2.70	1.93	
	Minimum	12.00	13.00	12.00	
	Maximum	154.00	152.00	154.00	
Age, years	Mean	64.02	63.67	63.84	0.760
	SEM	0.85	0.81	0.59	
	Minimum	27.00	29.00	27.00	
	Maximum	93.00	91.00	93.00	
BMI, kg/m^2	Mean	30.18	29.63	29.91	0.361
	SEM	0.43	0.42	0.30	
	Minimum	16.40	18.60	16.40	
	Maximum	58.30	64.10	64.10	
Sex, n (%)	Male	135 (62.50)	134 (66.20)	278 (64.35)	0.423
	Female	81 (37.50)	73 (33.80)	154 (35.65)	
Affected side, n (%)	Left	111 (51.39)	95 (43.98)	206 (47.69)	0.124
	Right	105 (48.61)	121 (56.02)	226 (52.32)	
Smoker, n (%)	Yes	51 (23.61)	34 (15.74)	85 (19.68)	0.029
	No	159 (73.61)	181 (83.80)	340 (78.70)	
	n.a.	6 (2.78)	1 (0.46)	7 (1.62)	
Pre-existing conditions (multiple answer), n (%)	Associated metabolic syndrome	82 (37.96)	79 (36.57)	161 (37.27)	0.385
	Rheumatism	10 (4.63)	8 (3.70)	18 (4.17)	
	Others	44 (20.37)	29 (13.43)	73 (16.90)	
	None	45 (20.83)	57 (26.51)	102 (23.61)	
Initial injury, (multiple answer), n (%)	Ankle fracture	120 (55.56)	134 (62.04)	254 (58.79)	0.054
	Ankle Ligament Tear	15 (6.94)	47 (21.76)	62 (14.35)	<0.001
	Syndesmotic injury	16 (7.41)	22 (10.18)	38 (8.79)	0.196
	Failure of Total Ankle Arthroplasty	29 (13.43)	9 (4.17)	38 (8.79)	0.003
	Talar fracture	24 (11.11)	6 (2.78)	30 (6.94)	<0.001
	Others	43 (19.9)	51 (23.61)	94 (21.76)	0.251

BMI, body mass index; SEM, standard error of the mean; TTC, Tibiotalocalcaneal Arthrodesis; TT, Tibiotalar Arthrodesis.

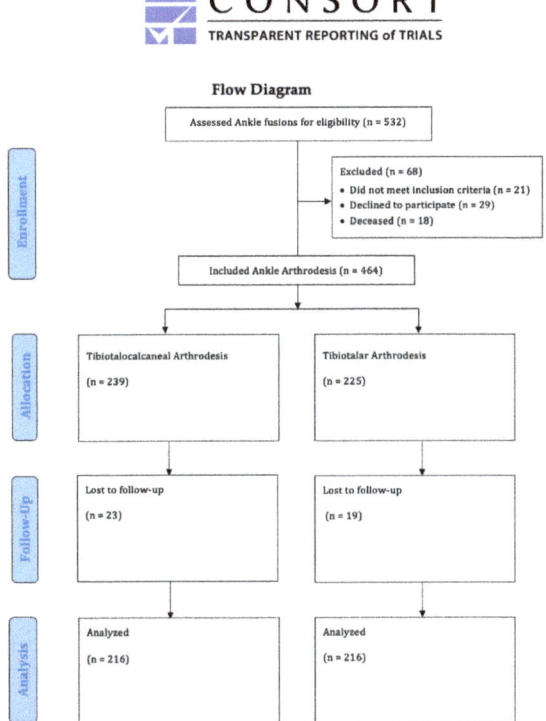

Figure 1. Study flow chart.

All patients underwent TTCA or TTA at the study center by five surgeons with the same expertise in this type of surgery. The mean follow-up duration for clinical outcomes was 6.2 years (range: 12–154 months). All procedures were performed in accordance with the 1964 Helsinki Declaration and its later amendments. The ethics committee of the institutional review board approved this study (2022-2883-evBO).

2.2. Inclusion and Exclusion Criteria

Patients older than 18 years were included; there was no maximum age limit. Written informed consent was required prior to participation. The indication for surgery was based on underlying painful end-stage posttraumatic osteoarthritis of the tibiotalar and additional subtalar joint leading to TTCA or TTA. Only surgeries performed at the study center were included. Destruction of the ankle joint due to rheumatic disease or malignant neoplasm of bone, such as osteosarcoma with multiple reconstructions and eventual tibiotalar fusion, were not included.

2.3. Surgical Procedures

The decision for TTCA or TTA on the basis of the objectifiable radiological criteria was largely guided by the surgeon's personal experience, the expected osteoarthritis of the subtalar joint, and the patient's expectations. Uniform criteria could only be completely delimited at follow-up. The surgical procedures were performed under general anesthesia or, less frequently, under spinal anesthesia, and a tourniquet was obligatorily applied to the thigh. The patient was placed in a supine position for both procedures.

For TTCA, the approach was usually along the lateral malleolus, which is osteotomized and decorticated 5–10 cm proximal to the tip of the malleolus, depending on the size of the patient and pre-ordered destruction of the ankle joint. The tibiotalar and subtalar joint was then dissected via this approach, with the removal of any remaining cartilage and resection of the destroyed subchondral sclerosis. All TTCAs were performed by implantation of a hindfoot fusion nail with 5° valgus. The diameter and length of the nail were chosen to be between 150 mm and 300 mm according to preoperative planning and intraoperative findings (Figure 2). A shorter nail with a diameter of 12 mm was the most common. Interposition autologous or allogenic cancellous bone grafting was performed in less than 20% of cases.

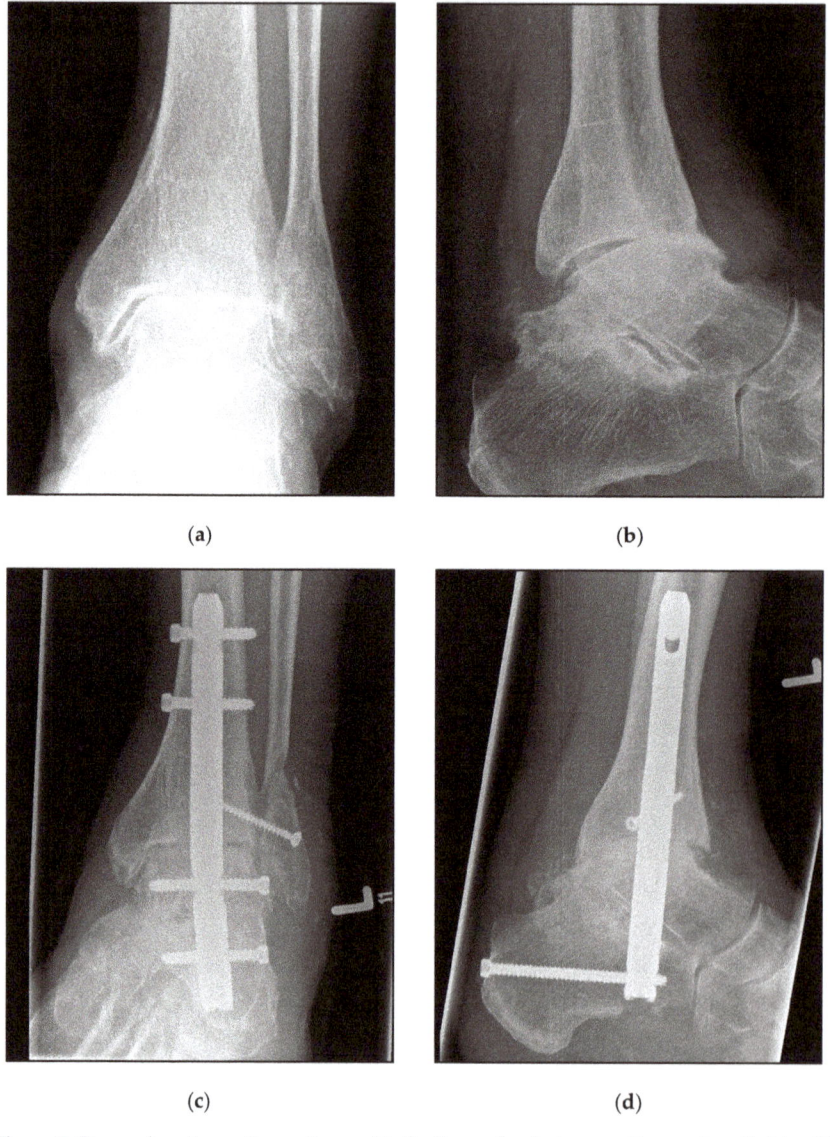

Figure 2. Pre- and postoperative radiographic findings of end-stage posttraumatic arthritis of the left ankle of a 79-year-old male treated with a tibiotalocalcaneal arthrodesis (TTCA) T2™ Ankle Arthrodesis Nail, 150 × 12 mm. (**a**,**b**) Anteroposterior view, preoperative. (**c**,**d**) Anteroposterior view, 3 months postoperative.

TTA was regularly performed via an anterior approach between the tibialis anterior and the extenso hallucis longus tendon. After the prescribed preparation of the joint, a fusion was performed by inserting 2–3 converging cannulated screws (diameter of 6.5 or 8 mm) or an anterior fusion plate (Figure 3). Other approaches, such as lateral, posterolateral, and medial, as well as combined approaches, were also used where necessary. Nevertheless, treatment via the anterior approach was the most common, at over 80%. Regardless of the technical implementation, both the TTCA and the TTA were designed to be neutral in both the coronal and the sagittal plane, with a physiological valgus of the hindfoot of 5°.

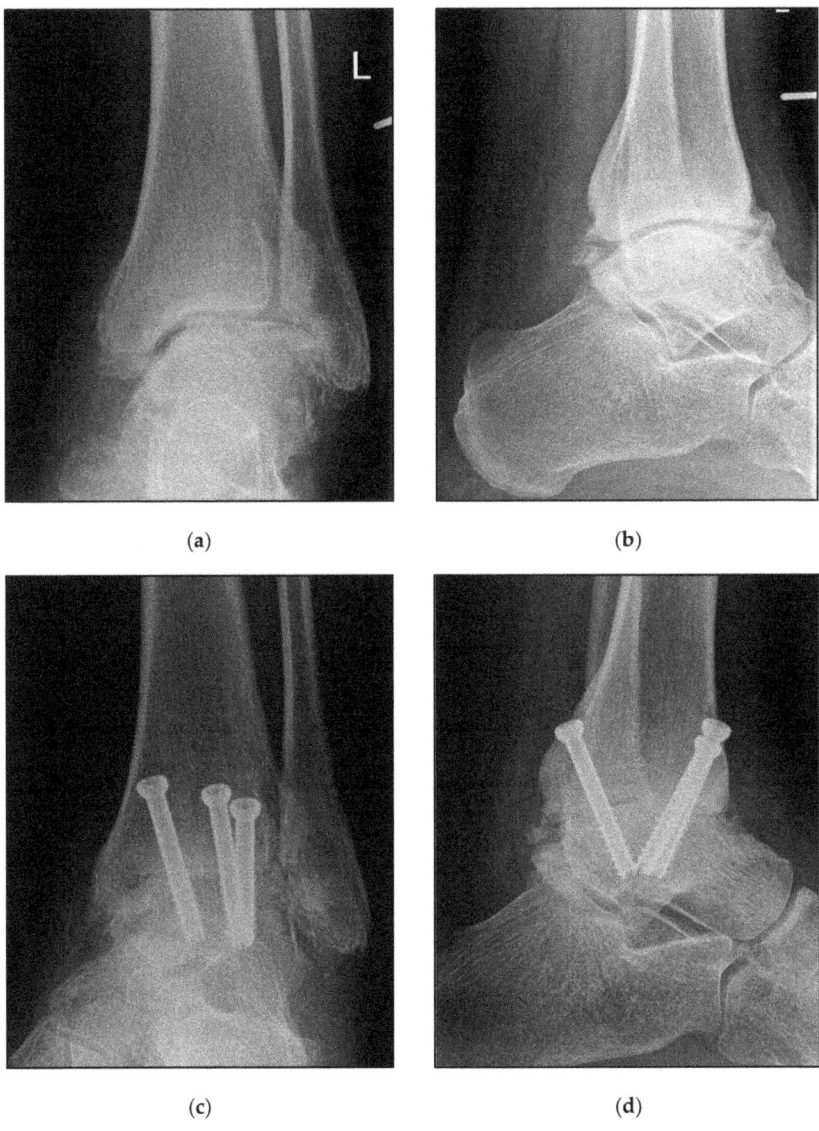

Figure 3. Pre- and postoperative radiographic findings of end-stage posttraumatic arthritis of the left ankle of a 44-year-old male treated with tibiotalar arthrodesis (TTA) using cannulated screws (diameter 6.5 mm). (a,b) Anteroposterior view, preoperative. (c,d) Anteroposterior view, 8 weeks postoperative.

2.4. Rehabilitation Protocol

The protocol following TTCA and TTA was the same. The post-treatment scheme involved wearing an orthotic boot (e.g., VACOped™) for a total of 12 weeks and ambulating on the forearm or armpit crutches. For the first 6 weeks, patients were required to wear the boot for 24 h a day with merely sole contact; removal of the boot for personal hygiene and physiotherapy was permitted.

After an X-ray examination, the boot was worn for an additional 6 weeks, with a gradual increase in load. During this time, the boot could be removed at night. At 12 weeks after surgery, computed tomography was carried out, and the footwear was orthopedically adapted for everyday use.

2.5. Assessment Methods

Demographic data, including age, body mass index (BMI), pre-existing conditions (such as those associated with syndrome-x), and nicotine abuse, were obtained for each patient. The Olerud & Molander Ankle Score (OMAS), Foot Function Index in its validated German version (FFI-D), the Short Form-12 Questionnaire (SF-12), and the type and number of revisions were recorded as part of the follow-up (Table 1).

2.6. Statistical Analysis

The primary goal was to compare significant differences in the outcome of TTCA and TTA using a representative number of patients to illustrate the power of the included data with a mean follow-up time of 6.2 years. Due to the retrospective design, there is no case number calculation. So far, monocentric studies with comparable questions have presented significantly smaller populations [7,8]. All statistical analyses were performed using SPSS v. 23 software (IBM Dtl. GmbH, Ehningen, Germany). Furthermore, descriptive and explorative statistical analyses for the queried scores, including within-group means, medians, minima and maxima, and standard deviations, were applied. Student's *t*-test and ANOVA were used. The power of the study was 0.8, and the significance level was set to $p < 0.05$, with a 95% confidence interval.

3. Results

After an average postoperative follow-up of 74 months (range: 12–154 months), the mean OMAS and FFI-D scores were 50.7 (TTCA: 43.0; TTA: 58.2) and 68.9 points, respectively. The difference was significant, as was the physical component summary of the SF-12 (mean: 39.1; TTCA: 33.5; TTA: 42.5), ($p < 0.001$).

The ability of the patient to return to their job also differed significantly: in the TTCA group, around 15% returned successfully; in the TTA group, 26% ($p < 0.001$). Only the mental component summary of the SF-12 showed no significant difference, with a mean value of 50.6 for all patients ($p = 0.369$). In a free survey, one-third of patients reported that their gait was as expected after the arthrodesis, one-third reported that it was worse, and one-third managed better than expected before surgery. The distribution applied equally to both groups.

Complications

The overall revision rate was approximately 19%, with a significantly higher proportion in the TTCA group (all $n = 80$; TTCA: $n = 64$ (29.6%), TTA: $n = 16$ (7.41%); $p < 0.001$). Most revisions had to be performed due to non-union and infections. In addition, minor complications, such as delayed wound healing, swelling, discomfort, and cramps, were recorded (Table 2).

Table 2. Clinical outcome with subgroups.

Measurements		TTCA (n = 216)	TTA (n = 216)	All (n = 432)	p
Olerud & Molander	Mean	43.00	58.16	50.67	<0.001
	SEM	1.68	1.67	1.24	
	Minimum	0.00	0.00	0.00	
	Maximum	100.00	100.00	100.00	
FFI-D	Mean	76.64	61.36	68.89	<0.001
	SEM	1.98	2.17	1.52	
	Minimum	15.00	5.00	5.00	
	Maximum	135.00	140.00	140.00	
SF-12 (Physical component summary)	Mean	35.52	42.49	39.07	<0.001
	SEM	0.75	0.71	0.54	
	Minimum	11.73	16.54	11.73	
	Maximum	56.63	61.22	61.22	
SF-12 (Mental component summary)	Mean	50.09	51.07	50.59	0.369
	SEM	0.81	0.72	0.54	
	Minimum	17.10	18.39	17.10	
	Maximum	68.89	71.03	71.03	
Gait after surgery as expected	As expected	80 (37.04)	83 (38.43)	163 (37.73)	0.360
	Better than expected	63 (29.17)	91 (42.13)	154 (35.65)	
	Worse than expected	63 (29.17)	40 (18.52)	103 (23.84)	
	n.a.	10 (4.63)	2 (0.93)	12 (2.78)	
Complication, Revision surgery needed (multiple answer), n (%)	Yes	64 (29.63)	16 (7.41)	80 (18.52)	<0.001
	No	152 (70.37)	200 (92.59)	352 (81.48)	
	Infection	23 (10.65)	5 (2.32)	28 (6.48)	<0.001
	Non-union	32 (14.81)	5 (2.32)	37 (8.57)	<0.001
Footwear (multiple answer), n (%)	Orthotic insoles only	41 (18.98)	72 (33.33)	113 (26.16)	0.002
	Shoe adaption	106 (49.07)	66 (30.56)	172 (39.82)	
	Others	9 (4.17)	2 (0.93)	11 (2.55)	
	Nothing special	60 (27.78)	76 (35.19)	136 (31.48)	
Return to the learned profession, n (%)	Yes	33 (15.28)	57 (26.39)	90 (20.83)	<0.001
Permanently unable to work, n (%)	Yes	49 (22.68)	26 (12.04)	75 (17.36)	<0.001
Retraining, part-time, pension, n (%)	Yes	134 (62.04)	133 (61.57)	267 (61.81)	>0.05

SEM, standard error of the mean; MT, metatarsal; SF-12, 12-Item Short Form Health Survey; TTCA, Tibiotalocalcaneal Arthrodesis; TTA, Tibiotalar Arthrodesis.

4. Discussion

TTCA and TTA for the treatment of end-stage posttraumatic osteoarthritis of the ankle yielded significant differences in our validated scores. If an additional subtalar arthrodesis is necessary, in addition to the pure tibiotalar arthrodesis, this represents a massive impairment of quality of life. These patients will elicit significantly poorer results compared to those undergoing isolated tibiotalar arthrodesis.

The aim of TTCA and TTA is the relief of pain caused by end-stage posttraumatic arthrosis, as well as to straighten possible malpositions and establish stability. Both methods are established in this regard. However, there is still no clear guideline as to which patients benefit from subtalar arthrodesis in the context of ankle fusion. Direct comparisons, especially in studies with a population with only terminal posttraumatic osteoarthritis of the ankle that is comparable in terms of risk profile and demographic data, only show the results of a small number of cases [7]. The results of TTCA and TTA vary from good for bone consolidation, reduced postoperative complications, and improvement of pain and quality of life, to the suggestion that additionally fusing the subtalar joint does not cause greater movement restriction [8–10]. Both these statements are difficult to understand on the basis of our data. Rather, we have confirmed that the subtalar joint plays a decisive role in mobility, especially in the case of an already fused tibiotalar joint. The additional requirement of a fusion of the subtalar joint leads to a considerable restriction of mobility with a corresponding reduction in quality of life. Regardless of this assessment, the results of the quality of life scores for TTCA and TTA reflect the respective results of the current literature without significant deviations [11–13].

Since no relevant differences could be determined from the subgroup analysis of the respective arthrodesis procedures in the TTA group, a separate presentation of the results was not carried out. This is in accordance with Prissel et al., who also showed no significant difference in clinical and radiological outcomes with similar complication rates after ankle arthrodesis using anterior locking plate fixation or converging screws [14]. Thus, the present data confirm the biomechanical and clinical studies that put the importance of the screw diameter and number into perspective [15]. In our procedures, two, three, or even four converging cannulated screws were inserted in the TTA group. An additional arthrodesis of the distal tibiofibular joint as part of the TTCA or TTA also showed no influence on the results and was carried out in about half of all cases. The clinical impression that simultaneous arthrodesis of the distal tibiofibular joint has no influence on the fusion rate of the tibiotalar joint and the further outcome was confirmed by Schlickewei et al. [16].

The interposition of cancellous bone also showed no influence on the data presented [17,18]. As a rule, there is no need for autologous cancellous bone grafting in the context of ankle arthrodesis, as confirmed by systematic reviews. As in the present case, the underlying studies lack a prospective comparison and, in the case of autologous cancellous bone grafting, an objectifiable representation of the previous bony defect size [18].

We also found that the mental component summary of SF-12 was the only parameter that did not show a significant difference ($p = 0.369$). An obvious explanation for this may be that patients in whom an additional fusion of the subtalar joint was necessary were assumed to have an even worse function. In addition, these patients presumably come from a worse initial function, but this cannot be evaluated on the basis of the available data. Either way, the results of the mental component summary of SF-12 of the present study deviate from those of the current literature in patients after TTCA, TTA, and even after total ankle replacement [10,19–21].

Even though the stated complication rates of 19% for TTCA and TTC remain high, these results differ considerably from those in the literature of up to a frightening 50% [22–24]. The complication rate for TTCA is approximately four times higher than that for TTA (30% vs. 7%, respectively). TTCA should, therefore, be considered with appropriate restraint. One conceivable explanation would be the higher proportion of smokers in the TTCA group. In addition, the procedure immanent greater soft tissue damage.

This study had some limitations. First, this was a monocentric study with a retrospective design and clinical scores and the extent of posttraumatic damage to the tibiotalar and subtalar joints was not collected preoperatively. This makes it particularly difficult to assess the choice of implant and the need for cancellous bone grafting. Second, the indication for TTCA and TTA was presumably influenced by surgeon experience.

5. Conclusions

Based on the present data of significantly worse clinical score results of TTCA compared to TTA, the fourfold complication rate, and the prolonged downtime and possible permanent incapacity, the indication for a generous subtalar joint arthrodesis with planned ankle arthrodesis should always be critically examined.

Author Contributions: Conceptualization, methodology, S.F. and M.M.; writing—original draft preparation, and writing—review and editing, R.S. and S.F.; software, validation, and formal analysis, A.K. and Y.G.; investigation and data curation, R.S. and O.N.; resources and supervision, E.H. and M.M.; project administration, R.H. and S.F. All authors have read and agreed to the published version of the manuscript.

Funding: This research received no external funding.

Institutional Review Board Statement: All procedures were performed in accordance with the 1964 Helsinki Declaration and its later amendments. This study was approved by the Institutional Review Board of the Hessian Medical Association Germany (2022-2883-evBO, 29 July 2022).

Informed Consent Statement: Informed consent was obtained from all subjects involved in the study. Written informed consent has been obtained from the patients to publish this paper.

Data Availability Statement: All data intended for publication are included in the manuscript.

Acknowledgments: Sincere thanks are extended to all co-authors for their excellent cooperation. No other grants were received.

Conflicts of Interest: The authors declare no conflict of interest.

References

1. Saltzman, C.L.; Salamon, M.L.; Blanchard, G.M.; Huff, T.; Hayes, A.; Buckwalter, J.A.; Amendola, A. Epidemiology of ankle arthritis: Report of a consecutive series of 639 patients from a tertiary orthopaedic center. *Iowa Orthop. J.* **2005**, *25*, 44–46. [PubMed]
2. Vitiello, R.; Perna, A.; Peruzzi, M.; Pitocco, D.; Marco, G. Clinical evaluation of tibiocalcaneal arthrodesis with retrograde intramedullary nail fixation in diabetic patients. *Acta Orthop. Traumatol. Turc.* **2020**, *54*, 255–261. [CrossRef] [PubMed]
3. Fischer, S.; Klug, A.; Faul, P.; Hoffmann, R.; Manegold, S.; Gramlich, Y. Superiority of upper ankle arthrodesis over total ankle replacement in the treatment of end-stage posttraumatic ankle arthrosis. *Arch. Orthop. Trauma Surg.* **2022**, *142*, 435–442. [CrossRef] [PubMed]
4. Watts, D.T.; Moosa, A.; Elahi, Z.; Palmer, A.J.R.; Rodriguez-Merchan, E.C. Comparing the Results of Total Ankle Arthroplasty vs. Tibiotalar Fusion (Ankle Arthrodesis) in Patients with Ankle Osteoarthritis since 2006 to 2020—A Systematic Review. *Arch. Bone Jt. Surg.* **2022**, *10*, 470–479. [CrossRef] [PubMed]
5. Easley, M.E.; Montijo, H.E.; Wilson, J.B.; Fitch, R.D.; Nunley, J.A., 2nd. Revision tibiotalar arthrodesis. *J. Bone Joint Surg. Am.* **2008**, *90*, 1212–1223. [CrossRef]
6. Cibura, C.; Lotzien, S.; Yilmaz, E.; Baecker, H.; Schildhauer, T.A.; Gessmann, J. Simultaneous septic arthrodesis of the tibiotalar and subtalar joints with the Ilizarov external fixator-an analysis of 13 patients. *Eur. J. Orthop. Surg. Traumatol.* **2022**, *32*, 1063–1070. [CrossRef]
7. Ajis, A.; Tan, K.J.; Myerson, M.S. Ankle arthrodesis vs. TTC arthrodesis: Patient outcomes, satisfaction, and return to activity. *Foot Ankle Int.* **2013**, *34*, 657–665. [CrossRef]
8. Cao, L.; Kyung, M.G.; Park, G.Y.; Hwang, I.U.; Kang, H.W.; Lee, D.Y. Foot and Ankle Motion after Tibiotalocalcaneal Arthrodesis: Comparison with Tibiotalar Arthrodesis Using a Multi-Segment Foot Model. *Clin. Orthop. Surg.* **2022**, *14*, 631–644. [CrossRef]
9. Perisano, C.; Cannella, A.; Polichetti, C.; Mascio, A.; Comisi, C.; De Santis, V.; Caravelli, S.; Mosca, M.; Spedicato, G.A.; Maccauro, G.; et al. Tibiotalar and Tibiotalocalcaneal Arthrodesis with Paragon28 Silverback(TM) Plating System in Patients with Severe Ankle and Hindfoot Deformity. *Medicina* **2023**, *59*, 344. [CrossRef]
10. Deleu, P.A.; Piron, M.; Leemrijse, G.; Besse, J.L.; Cheze, L.; Devos Bevernage, B.; Lalevee, M.; Leemrijse, T. Patients' point of view on the long-term results of total ankle arthroplasty, tibiotalar and tibiotalocalcaneal arthrodeses. *Orthop. Traumatol. Surg. Res.* **2022**, *108*, 103369. [CrossRef]
11. Lu, V.; Tennyson, M.; Zhang, J.; Thahir, A.; Zhou, A.; Krkovic, M. Ankle fusion with tibiotalocalcaneal retrograde nail for fragility ankle fractures: Outcomes at a major trauma centre. *Eur. J. Orthop. Surg. Traumatol.* **2023**, *33*, 125–133. [CrossRef] [PubMed]
12. Gowda, B.N.; Kumar, J.M. Outcome of ankle arthrodesis in posttraumatic arthritis. *Indian J. Orthop.* **2012**, *46*, 317–320. [CrossRef] [PubMed]
13. Maffulli, N.; Longo, U.G.; Locher, J.; Romeo, G.; Salvatore, G.; Denaro, V. Outcome of ankle arthrodesis and ankle prosthesis: A review of the current status. *Br. Med. Bull.* **2017**, *124*, 91–112. [CrossRef] [PubMed]
14. Prissel, M.A.; Simpson, G.A.; Sutphen, S.A.; Hyer, C.F.; Berlet, G.C. Ankle Arthrodesis: A Retrospective Analysis Comparing Single Column, Locked Anterior Plating to Crossed Lag Screw Technique. *J. Foot Ankle Surg.* **2017**, *56*, 453–456. [CrossRef]
15. Valiyev, N.; Demirel, M.; Hurmeydan, O.M.; Sunbuloglu, E.; Bozdag, E.; Kilicoglu, O. The Effects of Different Screw Combinations on the Initial Stability of Ankle Arthrodesis. *J. Am. Podiatr. Med. Assoc.* **2021**, *111*, 4. [CrossRef]
16. Schlickewei, C.; Neumann, J.A.; Yarar-Schlickewei, S.; Riepenhof, H.; Valderrabano, V.; Frosch, K.H.; Barg, A. Does Concurrent Distal Tibiofibular Joint Arthrodesis Affect the Nonunion and Complication Rates of Tibiotalar Arthrodesis? *J. Clin. Med.* **2022**, *11*, 3387. [CrossRef]
17. Gramlich, Y.; Neun, O.; Klug, A.; Buckup, J.; Stein, T.; Neumann, A.; Fischer, S.; Abt, H.P.; Hoffmann, R. Total ankle replacement leads to high revision rates in post-traumatic end-stage arthrosis. *Int. Orthop.* **2018**, *42*, 2375–2381. [CrossRef]
18. Heifner, J.J.; Monir, J.G.; Reb, C.W. Impact of Bone Graft on Fusion Rates in Primary Open Ankle Arthrodesis Fixated with Cannulated Screws: A Systematic Review. *J. Foot Ankle Surg.* **2021**, *60*, 802–806. [CrossRef]
19. Usuelli, F.G.; Pantalone, A.; Maccario, C.; Guelfi, M.; Salini, V. Sports and Recreational Activities following Total Ankle Replacement. *Joints* **2017**, *5*, 12–16. [CrossRef]

20. Rogero, R.G.; Fuchs, D.J.; Corr, D.; Shakked, R.J.; Raikin, S.M. Ankle Arthrodesis Through a Fibular-Sparing Anterior Approach. *Foot Ankle Int.* **2020**, *41*, 1480–1486. [CrossRef]
21. Yang, X.Q.; Zhang, Y.; Wang, Q.; Liang, J.Q.; Liu, L.; Liang, X.J.; Zhao, H.M. Supramalleolar Osteotomy vs. Arthrodesis for the Treatment of Takakura 3B Ankle Osteoarthritis. *Foot Ankle Int.* **2022**, *43*, 1185–1193. [CrossRef] [PubMed]
22. Cooper, P.S. Complications of ankle and tibiotalocalcaneal arthrodesis. *Clin. Orthop. Relat. Res.* **2001**, *391*, 33–44. [CrossRef] [PubMed]
23. Crosby, L.A.; Yee, T.C.; Formanek, T.S.; Fitzgibbons, T.C. Complications following arthroscopic ankle arthrodesis. *Foot Ankle Int.* **1996**, *17*, 340–342. [CrossRef] [PubMed]
24. Muir, D.C.; Amendola, A.; Saltzman, C.L. Long-term outcome of ankle arthrodesis. *Foot Ankle Clin.* **2002**, *7*, 703–708. [CrossRef]

Disclaimer/Publisher's Note: The statements, opinions and data contained in all publications are solely those of the individual author(s) and contributor(s) and not of MDPI and/or the editor(s). MDPI and/or the editor(s) disclaim responsibility for any injury to people or property resulting from any ideas, methods, instructions or products referred to in the content.

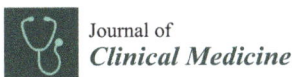

Journal of
Clinical Medicine

Article

In Vivo Foot Segmental Motion and Coupling Analysis during Midterm Follow-Up after the Open Reduction Internal Fixation of Trimalleolar Fractures

Harm Hoekstra [1,2,*], Olivier Vinckier [3,*], Filip Staes [4], Lisa Berckmans [4], Jolien Coninx [4], Giovanni Matricali [2,3,5], Sander Wuite [2,3,5], Eline Vanstraelen [6] and Kevin Deschamps [4,6,7,8]

[1] Department of Trauma Surgery, University Hospitals Leuven, Herestraat 49, 3000 Leuven, Belgium
[2] Department of Development and Regeneration, KU Leuven—University of Leuven, 3000 Leuven, Belgium
[3] Department of Orthopaedics, University Hospitals Leuven, Herestraat 49, 3000 Leuven, Belgium
[4] Musculoskeletal Rehabilitation Research Group, Department of Rehabilitation Sciences, KU Leuven—University of Leuven, Tervuursevest 101, 3001 Leuven, Belgium
[5] Institute for Orthopaedic Research and Training, KU Leuven—University of Leuven, Herestraat 49, 3000 Leuven, Belgium
[6] Clinical Motion Analysis Laboratory, Campus Pellenberg, University Hospitals Leuven, Weligerveld 1, 3212 Lubbeek, Belgium
[7] Division of Podiatry, Institut D'Enseignement Supérieur Parnasse Deux-Alice, Haute Ecole Leonard de Vinci, Avenue e Mounier 84, 1200 Bruxelles, Belgium
[8] Department of Podiatry, Artevelde University College, Hoogpoort 15, 9000 Gent, Belgium
* Correspondence: harm.hoekstra@uzleuven.be (H.H.); olivier.vinckier@gmail.com (O.V.)

Abstract: Purpose: Trimalleolar ankle fractures (TAFs) are common traumatic injuries. Studies have described postoperative clinical outcomes in relation to fracture morphology, but less is known about foot biomechanics, especially in patients treated for TAFs. The aim of this study was to analyze segmental foot mobility and joint coupling during the gait of patients after TAF treatment. Methods: Fifteen patients, surgically treated for TAFs, were recruited. The affected side was compared to their non-affected side, as well as to a healthy control subject. The Rizzoli foot model was used to quantify inter-segment joint angles and joint coupling. The stance phase was observed and divided into sub-phases. Patient-reported outcome measures were evaluated. Results: Patients treated for TAFs showed a reduced range of motion in the affected ankle during the loading response (3.8 ± 0.9) and pre-swing phase (12.7 ± 3.5) as compared to their non-affected sides (4.7 ± 1.1 and 16.1 ± 3.1) and the control subject. The dorsiflexion of the first metatarsophalangeal joint during the pre-swing phase was reduced (19.0 ± 6.5) when compared to the non-affected side (23.3 ± 8.7). The affected side's Chopart joint showed an increased range of motion during the mid-stance (1.3 ± 0.5 vs. 1.1 ± 0.6). Smaller joint coupling was observed on both the patient-affected and non-affected sides compared to the controls. Conclusion: This study indicates that the Chopart joint compensates for changes in the ankle segment after TAF osteosynthesis. Furthermore, reduced joint-coupling was observed. However, the minimal case numbers and study power limited the effect size of this study. Nevertheless, these new insights could help to elucidate foot biomechanics in these patients, adjusting rehabilitation programs, thereby lowering the risk of postoperative long-term complications.

Keywords: coupling analysis; foot segmental motion; trimalleolar ankle fractures

Citation: Hoekstra, H.; Vinckier, O.; Staes, F.; Berckmans, L.; Coninx, J.; Matricali, G.; Wuite, S.; Vanstraelen, E.; Deschamps, K. In Vivo Foot Segmental Motion and Coupling Analysis during Midterm Follow-Up after the Open Reduction Internal Fixation of Trimalleolar Fractures. *J. Clin. Med.* 2023, 12, 2772. https://doi.org/10.3390/jcm12082772

Academic Editors: Andreas Neff and Wing Hoi Cheung

Received: 19 February 2023
Revised: 31 March 2023
Accepted: 5 April 2023
Published: 7 April 2023

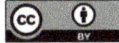

Copyright: © 2023 by the authors. Licensee MDPI, Basel, Switzerland. This article is an open access article distributed under the terms and conditions of the Creative Commons Attribution (CC BY) license (https:// creativecommons.org/licenses/by/ 4.0/).

1. Introduction

Ankle fractures are relatively common musculoskeletal injuries with an average incidence of 168.7/100,000/year [1]. The posterior tibia is involved in almost half of the Weber type B or C ankle fracture dislocations [2]. In most cases, a high-energy trauma is the primary cause of a trimalleolar ankle fracture (TAF), wherein both the medial, lateral, and posterior malleolus are involved. The trauma-mechanism-based Lauge–Hansen classification has been used for many years in guiding treatment and predicting instability. This system is built on a comprehensive understanding of trauma mechanism and the interplay between fracture morphology and ligamentous injury. The open reduction and internal fixation of the posterior malleolus, via either a posterolateral or posteromedial approach, is most commonly applied in our center for these fractures [3]. However, there is still a lack of consensus on whether the fixation of the posterior malleolus is always necessary. Treatment strategies that take the size and displacement of the posterior fracture fragment into consideration remain an issue of debate [4–6].

TAFs and subsequent plate osteosynthesis are associated with osteoarthritis, arthrofibrosis, and fibro-adhesions (i.e., flexor hallucis longus and peroneal muscles), leading to restriction in ankle joint mobility [7–10]. Subsequently, alterations in foot joint mobility, segment coupling (kinematic relationship between adjacent foot segments), and kinetics (forces acting on the foot joints) during gait may occur as well. It has been theorized that altered or disrupted coupling mechanisms may contribute to poor functional outcome scores due to pathological joint contact forces and soft tissue stress [11,12]. Nevertheless, there is a lack of in vivo dynamic assessments on the foot which specific focus on the functional outcomes of patients with a history of TAF osteosynthesis. Previous studies that reported on foot kinematics after the operative treatment of ankle fractures consisted of heterogeneous groups and used the Oxford foot model, which does not include the midfoot as a separate segment [13,14].

Therefore, we aimed to measure the segmental foot mobility and joint coupling of patients with a history of a TAF osteosynthesis. The affected side was compared to the non-affected contralateral side, as well as with a healthy control group. We hypothesized a reduction in the affected sides' hindfoot range of motion (ROM) during the loading response and the pre-swing of the stance phase, with most distinct changes seen in the frontal plane and sagittal plane, respectively. Furthermore, we hypothesized a reduced joint coupling between hindfoot and shank, as well as between the hindfoot and the forefoot.

2. Materials and Methods

Level of Evidence: III.

2.1. Patients

Fifteen patients who sustained a TAF (AO/OTA type B3) and underwent open reduction and internal fixation were retrospectively recruited. All patients underwent surgery between 2015 and 2018 at the Trauma Surgery department of the University Hospitals Leuven. Five patients had a luxation of the tibiotalar joint and two patients had a subluxation of the tibiotalar joint. None of the patient group had an open fracture. Polytrauma was not included in our study population. In total, 10 of the 15 patients obtained a temporary external fixator awaiting definitive internal fixation. The posterior malleolus and distal fibula fracture were addressed using plate screw osteosynthesis via a posterolateral approach, whereas the medial malleolus fracture was fixated using screws via a medial approach. Standardly one-third tubular plates with the small fragment system screws by DePuy Synthes™ (Raynham, MA, USA) were used to achieve anatomical reduction and internal fixation. If deemed necessary by the treating surgeon, variable angle LCP® was utilized in some cases. Additional syndesmotic screw fixation was performed if syndesmotic instability persisted after osseous fixation. Postoperatively, a fixed protocol was followed, consisting of immediate passive and active mobilization and toe-touch weight bearing (<10 kg) for 6 weeks. The control group consisted of 13 healthy subjects that were chosen at random from an existing database set-up in the same laboratory [6]. We matched a TAF subject to a control patient of the same gender, similar age, and walking speed to avoid the influence of confounding factors. An a priori sample size calculation showed that at least 12 patients and 12 control subjects were required to assure a minimal study power of 80% ($\beta > 0.80$). This calculation was based on biomechanical parameters reported in other studies, including patients with ankle osteoarthritis or ankle fractures [13,15]. Informed consent was obtained from all participants and the ethical committee of the University Hospitals Leuven (S62064) approved the study.

2.2. 3D Gait Analysis

In this study, a 3D gait analysis was performed in the Clinical Motion Analysis Laboratory of the University Hospitals Leuven Belgium. The analysis was performed using a multi-segment foot model where reflecting skin-markers were placed according to the Rizzoli foot model marker placement protocol using double-sided tape [16]. This multi-segment foot model calculates the 3D rotation between adjacent segments of the foot and tibia. For reasons of readability, these inter-segment angles will be reported with respect to their corresponding anatomical joints, i.e., the ankle segment (consisting of two joint levels: tibiotalar and subtalar), the Chopart joint, the Lisfranc joint, and the first metatarsophalangeal (MTP 1) joint. Kinematic data were captured with a passive optoelectronic measurement, including ten infrared cameras (T10, 100 Hz, Vicon Motion Systems Ltd., Oxford Metrics, UK). For this study, only the stance phase of gait was considered, which was delineated with initial contact as the start and toe-off as the end. The measurements were taken on the symptomatic side as well as the asymptomatic side. The first measurement was taken as a static recording and was used as a reference position. After this, the dynamic measurements were recorded. The participants were asked to repeatedly walk along a 10 m walkway at a self-selected speed until five representative trials were registered. The walkway was instrumented with a force plate (Advanced Mechanical Technology Inc., 200 Hz, Watertown, MA, USA) in order to determine the gait events such as the initial contact and the toe-off. A plantar pressure plate (Footscan™, dimensions 0.5 m × 0.4 m, 4096 sensors, 2.8 sensors per cm^2, RSscan International, Olen, Belgium) was placed on top of the force plate. Plantar pressure and force data were synchronized with a 3D box™ (RSscan International, Olen, Belgium) using an external trigger. These data were sampled at 200 Hz.

2.3. Data Processing and Analysis

The 3D inter-segment joint angles and joint coupling were calculated for the stance phase (0–62%) of the gait cycle. The swing phase of gait (63–100%) was not considered. In-house-made software (ACEPManager, Matlab 2016a, The Mathworks Inc., Natick, MA, USA) was used to normalize the time of the kinematic data to a 100% stance phase during the gait events. Kinematic variables of interest were subsequently calculated. We distinguished 4 sub-phases of the stance phase, i.e., the "loading response" (0–12%), "mid stance" (13–30%), "terminal stance" (31–50%), and "pre-swing" (51–62%) phases. Kinematic variables of interest were subsequently determined by calculating the ROM in each sub-phase. The latter was carried out by calculating the difference between the maximum and minimum value in the respective sub-phase. Furthermore, the patient-reported outcome measures, using the ankle–hindfoot scale (AOFAS), the EuroQol health scale (EQ-5D), and the EQ-5D visual analogue scale (VAS), were evaluated. The AOFAS monitors the progression of patients after foot and ankle surgery, the EQ-5D records the health state as rated by the caregiver, and the EQ-5D VAS assumes the individual's health state valuation [17,18].

2.4. Statistical Analysis

Statistical analysis was performed with SPSS Statistics 27.0 (IBM Corp., New York, NY, USA). When comparing the affected side to the non-affected side of the same subject, a test of normality, the Shapiro–Wilk test ($\alpha = 0.05$), was completed. For the variables that were not normally distributed, a Wilcoxon signed-rank test ($\alpha = 0.05$) was used to compare the samples. The other variables were statistically compared using a paired *t*-test t ($\alpha = 0.05$). A univariate analysis of variance (ANOVA) was used to compare the control group with the affected group. The same analysis was performed with the inclusion of the BMI as a covariate, since the BMIs of the patients were found to be significantly higher than those in the control group.

To guard against the inflation of a type I error but maintain statistical power across the multiple comparisons, an adjusted alpha level was applied by dividing the alpha level by the number of parameters ($p = 0.05/4 = 0.0125$). Additionally, the effect size was determined for each difference (Cohen's d for the *t*-tests, r for the Wilcoxon tests, and partial η^2 for the ANOVA tests). A large effect size can be interpreted when $d \geq 0.8$, $r \geq 0.5$, and $\eta^2 \geq 0.25$ [19,20].

To evaluate the level of joint coupling between a number of inter-segment angles, cross-correlation coefficients were calculated based on the 1D waveforms associated with the normalized stance phases [21]. The following four joint couplings were analyzed: ankle inversion–eversion with ankle adduction–abduction, ankle inversion–eversion with forefoot dorsal flexion–plantar flexion, ankle inversion–eversion with forefoot inversion–eversion, and ankle inversion–eversion with forefoot adduction–abduction. This selection was based on a previous publication, which showed the high correlation between these four inter-segment rotations [22]. When assessing the cross-correlation, the following benchmarks were used: a large joint coupling >0.7 or <−0.7, a medium joint coupling between (−) 0.3 and (−) 0.69, and a small joint coupling between −0.3 and 0.3 [22].

3. Results

3.1. Demographics

Demographic characteristics of the patient group and control group are presented in Table 1. The two groups had a similar age, length, and gender ratio. The walking speed did not differ significantly between the two groups. The TAF group had a significantly higher body mass index (BMI) compared to the control group ($p < 0.001$). The BMI was therefore considered as a confounding factor when analyzing the kinematic differences between these two groups. Gait analysis was performed for 29 months after surgery on average. Five patients were treated with a syndesmotic screw, because insufficient syndesmotic stability of the distal tibiofibular joint was achieved with the plate osteosynthesis of the posterior malleolus alone. The mean clinical follow-up lasted 101 weeks (range: 60–171). Seven of the fifteen patients underwent some kind of implant removal. One patient had a superficial wound infection after implant removal. One patient developed a chronic regional pain syndrome (CRPS). No non-unions or mal-unions were reported. Two patients showed progression towards tibiotalar osteoarthritis on the latest available X-rays.

Table 1. Baseline characteristics of participants.

	Patient Group (*n* = 15)	Control Group (*n* = 13)	*p*
Age (years)	54 (37–68)	47 (33–64)	0.037
Length (cm)	168.5 (151.0–190.3)	171.2 (158.0–193.3)	
Body mass (kg)	86.2 (58.6–120.3)	67.9 (54.0–95.0)	0.003
BMI (kg/m^2)	30.1 (22.9–37.7)	23.1 (19.5–26.6)	<0.001
Gender (male/female)	6/9	6/9	
Walking speed (m/s)	1.2 (1.0–1.4)	1.2 (1.0–1.4)	0.914
Months until post-surgical gait analysis	29 (8–49)		
Operative characteristics			
Side (L/R)	8/7		
Posterior plate fixation	15 (100%)		
Medial screw fixation	15 (100%)		
Fibula plate fixation	15 (100%)		
Syndesmotic screw	5 (33.3%)		

Continuous variables are expressed as means and ranges and categorical variables are presented as numbers and percentages. Abbreviations: L, left; R, right.

3.2. Patient-Reported Outcome Scores

The AOFAS, EQ-5D, and EQ-5D VAS scores are displayed in Table 2 with missing data for three patients [7]. The patients scored an average of 78 on the AOFAS survey, reflecting a good outcome after surgery (e.g., 100 = excellent score). For the first domain of the EQ-5D, mobility, the majority (67%) of the patient group (TAF) had moderate problems. None of the 12 patients reported self-care problems. The minority of patients (42%) suffered problems with daily activities, whereas two-thirds of the patients experienced moderate pain (67%). The presence of depression/anxiety was found to be negligible.

Table 2. Patient-reported outcomes after trimalleolar ankle fracture osteosynthesis.

	Patient Group ($n = 12$)
AOFAS score	78.3 (59.0–100)
EQ-5D score	
Mobility	
No problems	4 (33.3%)
Moderate problems	8 (66.7%)
Extreme problems	/
Self-care	
No problems	12 (100%)
Moderate problems	/
Extreme problems	/
Activities	
No problems	7 (58.3%)
Moderate problems	5 (41.7%)
Extreme problems	/
Pain/discomfort	
No problems	4 (33.3%)
Moderate problems	8 (66.7%)
Extreme problems	/
Depression/anxiety	
No problems	11 (91.7%)
Moderate problems	1 (8.3%)
Extreme problems	/
EQ-5D VAS	81.0 (50.0–100)

Categorical variables are expressed as numbers and percentages. The AOFAS is expressed as the mean and range. All questionnaires were standardized and tested for reproducibility and validated for the Dutch language. Three of the fifteen patients did not report their outcome scores. Abbreviations: AOFAS, American Orthopedic Foot and Ankle Society; EQ-5D, EuroQol 5 dimensions; VAS, visual analog scale.

3.3. ROM Comparisons of the Affected and Contralateral Side in the Patient Group

During the loading response, the ankle segment of the affected side presented a significantly reduced ROM in the sagittal plane ($p < 0.0125$, large effect) and a trend towards reduced frontal plane ROM ($p = 0.049$, medium effect) (Table 3, Figure 1). Furthermore, the Chopart joint of the affected foot showed a trend towards reduced frontal plane ROM during the loading response ($p = 0.013$) and a trend towards an increased ROM during the midstance phase ($p = 0.03$). No significant differences were observed during the terminal stance phase. During the pre-swing phase, the mean ankle segment sagittal and transverse plane ROM was significantly reduced ($p < 0.0125$) in the affected foot, with mean differences of $-3.4°$ and $-1.4°$ and effect sizes of $d = -0.9$ (large) and $d = -0.5$ (medium), respectively.

Table 3. Patient group ROM of the affected foot and non-affected contralateral sides.

			Affected Foot $n = 15$	Non-Affected Foot $n = 15$	Mean Difference [95% CI]	p	Effect Size
Loading response	Ankle	DF/PF	3.8 ± 0.9	4.7 ± 1.1	−0.9 [−1.6; −0.2]	0.010	−0.8
		Inv/Eve	2.9 ± 1.5	4.3 ± 1.9	−1.3 [−2.6; 0.0]	0.049	−0.6
		Add/Abd	1.3 ± 0.6	2.0 ± 1.2	−0.7 [−1.4; 0.1]	0.079	−0.5
	Chopart	DF/PF	1.8 ± 1.2	2.0 ± 1.3	−0.2 [−0.7; 0.3]	0.410	−0.2
		Inv/Eve	3.4 ± 0.9	4.3 ± 1.3	−0.8 [−1.5; −0.2]	0.013	−0.7
		Add/Abd	1.3 ± 0.9	1.2 ± 0.8	0.1 [−0.6; 0.8]	0.594	−0.1
	Lisfranc	PF/DF	3.6 ± 1.3	3.4 ± 1.5	0.2 [−0.6; 1.0]	0.551	−0.1
		Inv/Eve	1.8 ± 1.1	2.0 ± 1.1	−0.1 [−0.7; 0.5]	0.617	−0.1
		Add/Abd	2.5 ± 0.9	2.5 ± 1.1	0.0 [−0.7; 0.7]	0.970	−0.0
	MTP 1	DF/PF	8.0 ± 3.0	8.8 ± 7.0	−0.8 [−3.6; 1.9]	0.533	−0.2
Mid-stance	Ankle	DF/PF	5.2 ± 1.4	5.5 ± 1.6	−0.3 [−1.0; 0.3]	0.296	−0.3
		Inv/Eve	1.2 ± 0.6	1.6 ± 1.1	−0.4 [−1.1; 0.3]	0.683	−0.1
		Add/Abd	1.7 ± 1.3	2.3 ± 1.5	−0.6 [−1.4; 0.2]	0.109	−0.3
	Chopart	DF/PF	1.9 ± 0.7	2.0 ± 0.7	−0.1 [−0.5; 0.4]	0.707	−0.1
		Inv/Eve	1.3 ± 0.5	1.1 ± 0.6	0.3 [0.0; 0.5]	0.030	0.6
		Add/Abd	0.7 ± 0.5	0.7 ± 0.4	0.0 [−0.6; 0.6]	0.638	−0.1
	Lisfranc	DF/PF	1.2 ± 0.7	1.0 ± 0.6	0.2 [−0.4; 0.8]	0.510	0.1
		Inv/Eve	0.7 ± 0.5	0.7± 0.3	0.0 [−0.6; 0.6]	0.510	−0.1
		Add/Abd	1.1 ± 0.8	0.8 ± 0.6	0.3 [−0.4; 1.0]	0.140	−0.3
	MTP 1	DF/PF	4.0 ± 3.5	3.2 ± 2.5	0.8 [−0.1; 1.7]	0.778	−0.1
Terminal stance	Ankle	DF/PF	2.6 ± 1.2	2.5 ± 1.4	0.1 [−0.4; 0.7]	0.587	0.1
		Inv/Eve	3.6 ± 1.3	3.7 ± 1.4	−0.9 [−0.8; 0.7]	0.815	−0.1
		Add/Abd	3.7 ± 1.8	3.9 ± 1.8	−0.2 [−1.0; 0.6]	0.580	−0.1
	Chopart	DF/PF	5.5 ± 1.5	5.3 ± 1.6	0.2 [−0.6; 1.0]	0.582	0.1
		Inv/Eve	3.2 ± 1.2	2.8 ± 1.1	0.5 [−0.1; 1.0]	0.105	0.4
		Add/Abd	1.4 ± 0.7	1.3 ± 0.6	0.1 [−0.4; 0.7]	0.592	0.1
	Lisfranc	DF/PF	3.2 ± 1.3	3.5 ± 1.1	−0.3 [−1.0; 0.4]	0.177	−0.2
		Inv/Eve	1.9 ± 0.9	1.9 ± 1.0	0.0 [−0.6; 0.6]	0.992	0.0
		Add/Abd	2.6 ± 1.9	2.4 ± 1.4	0.3 [−0.5; 1.1]	0.465	0.2
	MTP 1	DF/PF	11.7 ± 4.8	11.7 ± 5.7	−0.1 [−2.3; 2.2]	0.960	−0.0
Pre-swing	Ankle	DF/PF	12.7 ± 3.5	16.1 ± 3.1	−3.4 [−5.6; −1.3]	0.004	−0.9
		Inv/Eve	2.3 ± 1.5	3.0 ± 1.6	−0.7 [−1.5; 0.1]	0.211	−0.2
		Add/Abd	2.3 ± 1.5	3.7 ± 2.9	−1.4 [−2.3; −0.5]	0.011	−0.5
	Chopart	DF/PF	9.5 ± 2.1	9.7 ± 2.6	−0.2 [−1.2; 0.9]	0.750	−0.1
		Inv/Eve	3.4 ± 1.8	3.4 ± 1.7	0.0 [−0.9; 0.8]	0.931	−0.0
		Add/Abd	3.1 ± 1.6	3.6 ± 2.1	−0.4 [−1.5; 0.7]	0.426	−0.2
	Lisfranc	DF/PF	4.5 ± 1.8	4.5 ± 1.8	0.0 [−0.8; 0.8]	0.470	−0.1
		Inv/Eve	2.1 ± 1.4	2.4 ± 1.7	−0.3 [−1.1; 0.5]	0.820	−0.0
		Add/Abd	5.9 ± 2.5	5.8 ± 3.1	0.1 [−1.2; 1.4]	0.836	0.1
	MTP 1	DF/PF	19.0 ± 6.5	23.3 ± 8.7	−4.5 [−8.5; −0.4]	0.040	−0.6

p values represent the outcome of the paired t-test ($\alpha = 0.05$); significance: $p < 0.0125$; when data were not normally distributed, the p values represent the outcome of the Wilcoxon test. Effect size represents the Cohen's d calculated for the t-test and r-value for the Wilcoxon test. Abbreviations: MTP 1, first metatarsophalangeal joint; DF/PF, dorsal flexion–plantar flexion (sagittal plane); Inv/Eve, inversion–eversion (frontal plane); Add/Abd, adduction–abduction (transverse plane).

3.4. Comparison ROM Affected Side in the Patient Group versus Control Group

During the loading response, the transverse plane ankle segment ROM was significantly ($p < 0.0125$) lower in the affected side (1.3 ± 0.6) compared to the control group (3.1 ± 1.1), with a large effect ($\eta^2 = 0.37$) (Table 4, Figure 1). During the midstance phase, the affected foot showed a reduced transverse plane ROM at the Chopart joint; hence, this did not reach a significance level. During the terminal stance phase, the affected foot demonstrated a reduced (p = 0.045) sagittal plane ROM at the ankle segment and an increased ROM in the Chopart joint (p = 0.038).

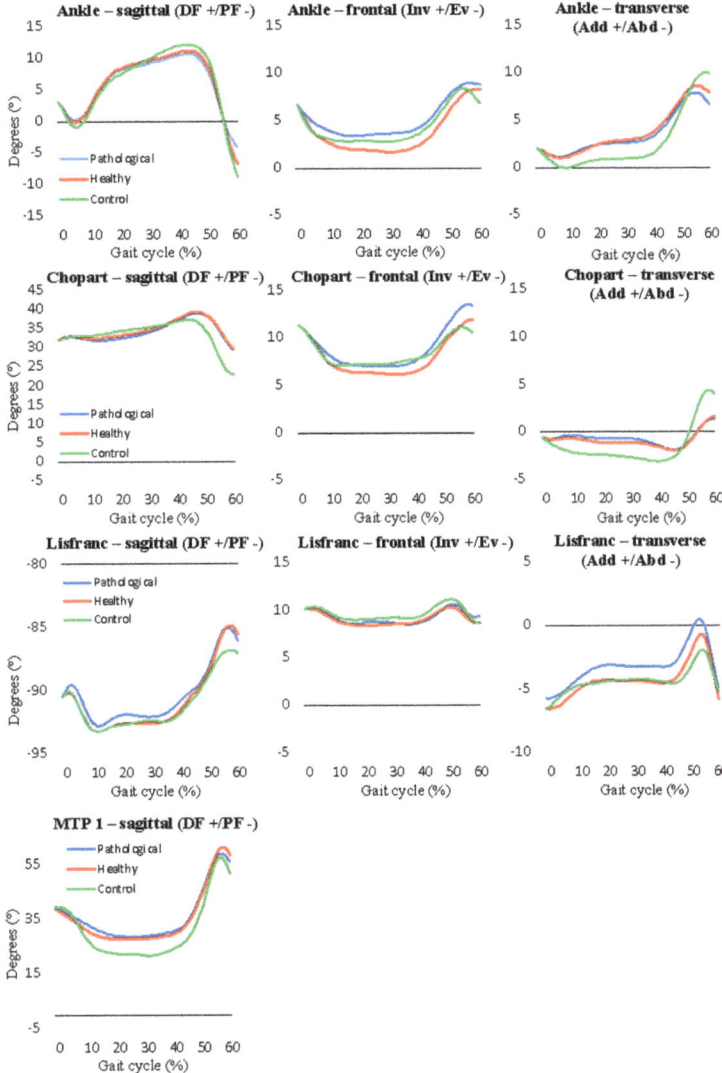

Figure 1. Kinematic waveforms of the ankle, Chopart, Lisfranc, and MTP 1 joints. Abbreviations: DF, dorsal flexion; PF, plantar flexion; Inv, inversion; Ev, eversion; Add, adduction; Abd, abduction.

During the pre-swing phase, the affected foot demonstrated a significantly reduced transverse plane ROM compared to the control group (p = 0.011, medium effect). Moreover, a clear trend towards reduced ROM was observed in other joints (ankle segment and Chopart joint) and planes (sagittal and transverse) as well.

Table 4. ROM of the affected foot versus the control group.

			Affected Foot	Controls	Mean Difference		
			n = 15	n = 13	[95% CI]	p	Partial η²
Loading response	Ankle	DF/PF	3.8 ± 0.9	5.1 ± 1.6	−1.3 [−2.1; −0.5]	0.096	0.11
		Inv/Eve	2.9 ± 1.5	3.9 ± 1.5	−0.9 [−1.7; −0.1]	0.872	0.00
		Add/Abd	1.3 ± 0.6	3.1 ± 1.1	−1.8 [−2.5; −1.1]	0.001	0.37
	Chopart	DF/PF	1.8 ± 1.2	3.1 ± 4.4	−1.3 [−2.2; −0.4]	0.539	0.02
		Inv/Eve	3.4 ± 0.9	4.4 ± 2.3	−1.0 [−1.8; −0.2]	0.172	0.07
		Add/Abd	1.3 ± 0.9	2.6 ± 2.8	−1.3 [−2.2; −0.4]	0.150	0.08
	Lisfranc	DF/PF	3.6 ± 1.3	3.6 ± 1.7	0.0 [−0.8; 0.8]	0.378	0.03
		Inv/Eve	1.8 ± 1.1	2.3 ± 1.2	−0.4 [−1.2; 0.4]	0.586	0.01
		Add/Abd	2.5 ± 0.9	2.3 ± 1.2	0.2 [−0.6; 1.0]	0.647	0.01
	MTP 1	DF/PF	8.0 ± 3.0	12.6 ± 10.1	−4.6 [−5.8; −3.4]	0.525	0.02
Midstance	Ankle	DF/PF	5.2 ± 1.4	6.1 ± 2.0	−1.0 [−1.8; −0.2]	0.167	0.08
		Inv/Eve	1.2 ± 0.6	1.2 ± 0.8	0.0 [−0.7; 0.7]	0.520	0.02
		Add/Abd	1.7 ± 1.3	1.8 ± 1.0	−0.1 [−0.9; 0.7]	0.960	0.00
	Chopart	DF/PF	1.9 ± 0.7	2.1 ± 2.0	−0.2 [−1.0; 0.6]	0.227	0.06
		Inv/Eve	1.3 ± 0.5	1.1 ± 0.6	0.2 [−0.4; 0.8]	0.469	0.02
		Add/Abd	0.7 ± 0.5	1.0 ± 0.5	0.3 [−0.3; 0.9]	0.048	0.15
	Lisfranc	DF/PF	1.2 ± 0.7	1.5 ± 1.0	0.2 [−0.5; 0.9]	0.274	0.05
		Inv/Eve	0.7 ± 0.5	0.7 ± 0.4	0.0 [−0.6; 0.6]	0.841	0.00
		Add/Abd	1.1 ± 0.8	1.0 ± 0.6	0.1 [−0.6; 0.8]	0.760	0.00
	MTP 1	DF/PF	4.0 ± 3.5	5.5 ± 2.2	−1.5 [−2.5; −0.5]	0.062	0.14
Terminal stance	Ankle	DF/PF	2.6 ± 1.2	3.6 ± 1.1	−1.0 [−1.8; −0.2]	0.045	0.15
		Inv/Eve	3.6 ± 1.3	3.8 ± 1.2	−0.2 [−1.0; 0.6]	0.765	0.00
		Add/Abd	3.7 ± 1.8	4.5 ± 2.5	−0.9 [−1.8; 0.0]	0.633	0.01
	Chopart	DF/PF	5.5 ± 1.5	3.1 ± 1.3	2.3 [1.5; 3.1]	0.038	0.16
		Inv/Eve	3.2 ± 1.2	2.7 ± 1.5	0.6 [−0.2; 1.4]	0.116	0.10
		Add/Abd	1.4 ± 0.7	2.1 ± 1.0	−0.6 [−1.3; 0.1]	0.088	0.11
	Lisfranc	DF/PF	3.2 ± 1.3	3.5 ± 1.3	−0.4 [−1.2; 0.4]	0.828	0.00
		Inv/Eve	1.9 ± 0.9	2.3 ± 1.1	−0.3 [−1.0; 0.4]	0.514	0.02
		Add/Abd	2.6 ± 1.9	2.5 ± 1.1	0.2 [−0.6; 1.0]	0.137	0.09
	MTP 1	DF/PF	11.7 ± 4.8	13.3 ± 5.6	−1.7 [−2.8; −0.6]	0.198	0.07
Pre-swing	Ankle	DF/PF	12.7 ± 3.5	19.4 ± 6.1	−6.7 [−7.8; −5.6]	0.025	0.19
		Inv/Eve	2.3 ± 1.5	2.6 ± 1.5	−0.3 [−1.1; 0.5]	0.334	0.04
		Add/Abd	2.3 ± 1.5	4.8 ± 2.6	−2.5 [−3.4; −1.6]	0.011	0.23
	Chopart	DF/PF	9.5 ± 2.1	12.9 ± 4.1	−3.4 [−4.4; −2.4]	0.033	0.17
		Inv/Eve	3.4 ± 1.8	2.8 ± 1.7	0.6 [−0.3; 1.5]	0.969	0.00
		Add/Abd	3.1 ± 1.6	5.9 ± 3.2	−2.7 [−3.6; −1.8]	0.028	0.18
	Lisfranc	DF/PF	4.0 ± 1.8	3.3 ± 2.2	0.8 [−0.1; 1.7]	0.111	0.10
		Inv/Eve	2.1 ± 1.4	3.1 ± 1.9	−1.0 [−1.8; −0.2]	0.203	0.06
		Add/Abd	5.9 ± 2.5	4.2 ± 1.8	1.7 [0.8; 2.6]	0.060	0.13
	MTP 1	DF/PF	19.0 ± 6.6	23.2 ± 11.1	−4.2 [−5.5; −2.9]	0.333	0.04

p values represent the outcomes of the one-way ANOVA test. BMI had no significant effect except a trend towards significance for Lisfranc Inv/Eve during pre-swing ($p = 0.035$); significance: $p < 0.0125$, trend to significance. Abbreviations: MTP 1, first metatarsophalangeal joint; DF/PF, dorsal flexion–plantar flexion (sagittal plane); Inv/Eve, inversion–eversion (frontal plane); Add/Abd, adduction–abduction (transverse plane).

3.5. Comparison Joint Coupling for the Three Cohorts

The cross-correlation coefficients showed a small joint coupling for the patient group in both feet when compared to the control group (Table 5). The largest differences were seen for the following inter-segment rotations: ankle inversion–eversion with ankle adduction–abduction, ankle inversion–eversion with forefoot dorsiflexion–plantarflexion, and ankle inversion–eversion with forefoot inversion–eversion. For these inter-segment rotations, the patient group showed a medium joint coupling ((−) 0.3 to (−) 0.69) for the non-affected and affected side, while the control group showed large joint coupling (>0.7 or <−0.7).

Table 5. Cross-correlation for all three cohorts.

	Contralateral Side	Affected Foot	Control Group
Ankle Inv/Eve–Ankle Add/Abd	0.623 ± 0.3	0.569 ± 0.2	0.873 ± 0.1
Ankle Inv/Eve–Forefoot DF/PF	−0.689 ± 0.3	−0.684 ± 0.2	−0.901 ± 0.1
Ankle Inv/Eve–Forefoot Inv/Eve	−0.666 ± 0.2	−0.634 ± 0.2	−0.791 ± 0.3
Ankle Inv/Eve–Forefoot Add/Abd	−0.118 ± 0.5	−0.135 ± 0.5	−0.147 ± 0.5

Abbreviations: DF/PF, dorsal flexion–plantar flexion (sagittal plane); Inv/Eve, inversion–eversion (frontal plane); Add/Abd, adduction–abduction (transverse plane).

4. Discussion

In this study, the segmental ROM and coupling of the foot joints were compared between patients that were operatively treated for a TAF and a control group. Only two previous studies have reported on foot kinematics after the operative treatment of ankle fractures. However, the patient cohorts were heterogeneous and the used Oxford foot model did not include the midfoot as a separate segment [13,14]. Moreover, both studies investigated coupling among the different segments of the foot.

In our study, we observed a general trend towards reduced ROM and joint coupling of the affected foot, particularly the ankle segment and midfoot joints. The patient group presented a mean body mass index corresponding to obesity class I, which is an interesting finding. From a functional viewpoint, it is reasonable to assume that an elevated BMI can be considered as a risk factor for moderate and low impact trauma, as frequently seen in TAFs. Nevertheless, further large-scale population studies are necessary to validate this assumption.

General information provided by the AOFAS score leads to the conclusion that the patients included in the population faced moderate pain and mobility problems at the onset of the investigation. The biomechanical outcome measures quantified here could thus also be (partly) explained by these patient' reported outcome measurements.

When comparing the patients' affected side to the contralateral non-affected side, some differences were obvious. The changes observed in the ankle segment during the loading response and the pre-swing phase can be a result of possible arthritis and arthro-fibrosis of the ankle joint and fibro-adhesions (i.e., muscle adhesions) due to surgery, which all affect ankle joint mobility [7–10]. Additionally, the involvement of pain at the affected foot may also contribute to the reduced ROM seen during the loading response and the pre-swing phase. The reduced ROM during the pre-swing phase may originate from the weakness of the calf muscles on the one hand, but could also be associated with a (mal)adaptive strategy of the patient in order to avoid peak loading in the posterior part of the ankle joint.

The Chopart joint of the affected foot had a significantly reduced ROM in the frontal plane during the loading response. A similar observation has been reported by Eerdekens et al. in patients with ankle osteoarthritis. This tibiotalar stiffness leads to the conclusion that this reduced motion is possibly associated with co-contraction and a more cautious walking strategy [23].

During the pre-swing phase, the MTP 1 joint of the affected foot showed a reduced ROM (mainly dorsal flexion) (Table 3 and Figure 1). This restriction may consequently be caused by muscle adhesions (fibro-adhesions) of the flexor hallucis longus muscle due to posterior plate osteosynthesis. However, from a functional viewpoint, this finding may also highlight a suboptimal usage of the "windlass mechanism" during propulsion, which in turn may affect the physiological joint coupling among the joints of the foot [24].

When comparing the affected foot of the patient group to the control group, a significant reduced transverse plane ankle ROM was quantified during the loading response. The latter observation explains the medium joint coupling observed between ankle inversion–eversion and adduction–abduction. Potential causes for this medium joint coupling may be due to arthro-fibrosis and fibro-adhesions at the posterior aspect of the ankle, the presence of co-contraction of extrinsic foot muscles, or alterations in foot placement during initial contact.

Differences in the ROM were also observed in the ankle segment and Chopart joint during the midstance, terminal stance, and pre-swing phases. Therefore, it can be concluded that there is less plantar flexion during propulsion in these joints (Figure 1) and the hindfoot tends to maintain a more abducted position. A similar observation was reported in the previous study of van Hoeve et al. [13]. Such a reduced plantar flexion was also observed when comparing the affected foot with the unaffected foot, which seems to point towards the presence of weakness of the calf muscles on the one hand or the presence of a (mal)adaptive strategy, avoiding any peak loading in the posterior aspect of the talus and posterior malleolus.

In the current study, small joint coupling was observed in the affected foot. One may hypothesize that this could be caused by perturbed neuromuscular control, proprioception, or the presence of arthro-fibrosis and muscle adhesions at the posterior aspect of the ankle. Despite the fact that these assumptions are realistic and logic, it should be recognized that a similar level of joint coupling was observed in the non-affected side of the patient group. This was an unexpected finding in the study and raises two new hypotheses. The first concerns whether the unaffected limb adopts a (mal)adaptive movement pattern to strive for gait symmetry. This adaptation is also seen in the knee after ACL reconstruction, where kinematic differences between the ACL-reconstructed limb and contralateral unaffected limb decrease over time because of alterations in both limbs [25]. A second hypothesis proposes that this smaller joint coupling was a pre-existing biomechanical phenomenon prior to the ankle trauma and that, together with the increased body mass, it can be considered as a risk factor for the development of ankle fractures. Further research is needed validate to validate or reject this hypothesis.

The postoperative rehabilitation for patients treated for a TAF needs to place emphasis on regaining full ankle joint mobility with passive and active exercises, as well as early protective weight bearing. Full plantar flexion mobility should be highlighted and transferred into the gait pattern, with a focus on the pre-swing phase. Gait training is thereby an important aspect of rehabilitation. Previous studies have concluded that early postoperative mobilization and weight bearing is safe and does not increase the complication rate in patients treated for ankle fractures [26–28]. Combining these aspects with weight reduction could lower the risk of developing post-traumatic osteoarthritis. Patients need to receive a home exercise program so that daily practice is possible and the patient can be autonomous in their treatment.

An important limitation of the current study is the non-standardized period between surgery and gait analysis. Within the patient group, the range was between 8 and 49 months after the operation. The differences in time between both events will influence the collected data because of dissimilarities in the recovery time. In addition, the low case numbers and the minimal study power result in limited practical applications. Another limitation is the condition of barefoot walking when the data were collected. When wearing shoes, the kinematic data may differ from the data during barefoot walking [29]. Lastly, this study only observed patients during walking. Therefore, these outcomes are not representable for more challenging tasks, e.g., running or jumping. It is hypothesized that more complex and challenging tasks may unravel other biomechanical differences than those reported here.

5. Conclusions

This study found that patients with a history of a TAF show reduced ROM in the affected ankle segment during the loading response and the pre-swing phase compared to their non-affected side and control subject. The affected sides' Chopart joint showed increased ROM during midstance to compensate for reduced ankle segment ROM during loading responses. Finally, small joint coupling was observed in the affected side as well as the non-affected side compared to the control group. Despite the limited effect size of our results, the findings of this study emphasize the importance of adequate postoperative rehabilitation to restore mobility and thereby potentially lower the risk of post-traumatic osteoarthritis in patients with a history of TAFs.

Author Contributions: H.H., O.V. and F.S. participated in the design and drafting of the manuscript; L.B. and J.C. collected the data and designed the manuscript; G.M. and S.W. helped to coordinate and draft the manuscript; E.V. participated in the sequence alignment; and K.D. conceived of the study, participated in its design and coordination, and helped to draft the manuscript. All authors have read and agreed to the published version of the manuscript.

Funding: This study was funded by the Belgian Society of Orthopedics and Traumatology (BVOT) with a EUR 4400 grant.

Institutional Review Board Statement: This study was completed in compliance with national legislation and the guidelines of the ethics committee of the University Hospitals Leuven (S62064). The study was conducted in accordance with the Declaration of Helsinki and approved by the Institutional Ethics Committee.

Informed Consent Statement: Informed consent was obtained from all subjects involved in the study.

Data Availability Statement: Not applicable.

Conflicts of Interest: The authors declare that they have no conflict of interest.

References

1. Elsoe, R.; Ostgaard, S.E.; Larsen, P. Population-based epidemiology of 9767 ankle fractures. *Foot Ankle Surg.* **2018**, *24*, 34–39. [CrossRef]
2. Jehlicka, D.; Bartonicek, J.; Svatos, F.; Dobias, J. Fracture-dislocations of the ankle joint in adults. Part I: Epidemiologic evaluation of patients during a 1-year period. *Chir. Orthop. Et Traumatol. Cechoslov.* **2022**, *69*, 243–247.
3. Hoekstra, H.; Rosseels, W.; Rammelt, S.; Nijs, S. Direct fixation of fractures of the posterior pilon via a posteromedial approach. *Injury* **2017**, *48*, 1269–1274. [CrossRef] [PubMed]
4. Xie, W.; Lu, H.; Zhan, S.; Liu, Y.; Xu, H.; Fu, Z.; Zhang, D.; Jiang, B. Outcomes of posterior malleolar fractures with intra-articular impacted fragment. *Arch. Orthop. Trauma Surg.* **2021**, *143*, 141–147. [CrossRef] [PubMed]
5. Verhage, S.M.; Hoogendoorn, J.M.; Krijnen, P.; Schipper, I.B. When and how to operate the posterior malleolus fragment in trimalleolar fractures: A systematic literature review. *Arch. Orthop. Trauma Surg.* **2018**, *138*, 1213–1222. [CrossRef]
6. Blom, R.P.; Hayat, B.; Al-Dirini RM, A.; Sierevelt, I.; Kerkhoffs GM, M.J.; Goslings, J.C.; Jaarsma, R.L.; Doornberg, J.N. Posterior malleolar ankle fractures: Predictors of outcome. *Bone Jt. J.* **2020**, *102*, 1229–1241. [CrossRef] [PubMed]
7. Mertens, M.; Wouters, J.; Kloos, J.; Nijs, S.; Hoekstra, H. Functional outcome and general health status after plate osteosynthesis of posterior malleolus fractures—The quest for eligibility. *Injury* **2020**, *51*, 1118–1124. [CrossRef] [PubMed]
8. Macera, A.; Carulli, C.; Sirleo, L.; Innocenti, M. Postoperative complications and reoperation rates following open reduction and internal fixation of ankle fracture. *Joints* **2018**, *6*, 110–115. [CrossRef]
9. Leyes, M.; Torres, R.; Guillén, P. Complications of open reduction and internal fixation of ankle fractures. *Foot Ankle Clin.* **2003**, *8*, 131–147. [CrossRef]
10. Caravelli, S.; Ambrosino, G.; Vocale, E.; Di Ponte, M.; Puccetti, G.; Perisano, C.; Greco, T.; Rinaldi, V.G.; Marcheggiani Muccioli, G.M.; Zaffagnini, S.; et al. Custom-Made Implants in Ankle Bone Loss: A Retrospective Assessment of Reconstruction/Arthrodesis in Sequelae of Septic Non-Union of the Tibial Pilon. *Medicina* **2022**, *58*, 1641. [CrossRef] [PubMed]
11. DeLeo, A.T.; Dierks, T.A.; Ferber, R.; Davis, I.S. Lower extremity joint coupling during running: A current update. *Clin. Biomech.* **2004**, *19*, 983–991. [CrossRef]
12. Ferber, R.; Hreljac, A.; Kendall, K.D. Suspected mechanisms in the cause of overuse running injuries: A clinical review. *Sports Health* **2009**, *1*, 242–246. [CrossRef] [PubMed]
13. Van Hoeve, S.; Houben, M.; Verbruggen JP, A.M.; Willems, P.; Meijer, K.; Poeze, M. Gait analysis related to functional outcome in patients operated for ankle fractures. *J. Orthop. Res.* **2019**, *37*, 1658–1666. [CrossRef]

14. Wang, R.; Thur, C.K.; Gutierrez-Farewik, E.M.; Wretenberg, P.; Broström, E. One year follow-up after operative ankle fractures: A prospective gait analysis study with a multi-segment foot model. *Gait Posture* **2010**, *31*, 234–240. [CrossRef] [PubMed]
15. Eerdekens, M.; Staes, F.; Matricali, G.A.; Wuite, S.; Peerlinck, K.; Deschamps, K. Quantifying clinical misinterpretations associated to one-segment kinetic foot modelling in both a healthy and patient population. *Clin. Biomech.* **2019**, *67*, 160–165. [CrossRef] [PubMed]
16. Leardini, A.; Benedetti, M.G.; Berti, L.; Bettinelli, D.; Nativo, R.; Giannini, S. Rear-foot, mid-foot and fore-foot motion during the stance phase of gait. *Gait Posture* **2007**, *25*, 453–462. [CrossRef]
17. De Boer, A.S.; Meuffels, D.E.; Van der Vlies, C.H.; Den Hoed, P.T.; Tuinebreijer, W.E.; Verhofstad, M.H.J.; Van Lieshout, E.M.M.; AOFAS Study Group. Validation of the American Orthopaedic Foot and Ankle Society Ankle-Hindfoot Scale Dutch language version in patients with hindfoot fractures. *BMJ Open* **2017**, *7*, e018314. [CrossRef]
18. Hung, M.C.; Lu, W.S.; Chen, S.S.; Hou, W.H.; Hsieh, C.L.; Wang, J.D. Validation of the EQ-5D in Patients with Traumatic Limb Injury. *J. Occup. Rehabil.* **2015**, *25*, 387–393. [CrossRef] [PubMed]
19. Cohen, J.; Cohen, P.; West, S.; Alken, L. *Applied Multiple Regression/Correlation Analysis for the Behavioral Sciences*; Routledge: Abingdon, UK, 2013; 736p.
20. Portney, L.; Watkins, M. *Foundations of Clinical Research Applications to Practice*, 3rd ed.; Pearson/Prentice Hall: Upper Saddle River, NJ, USA, 2014; 842p.
21. Li, L.; Caldwell, G.E. Coefficient of cross correlation and the time domain correspondence. *J. Electromyogr. Kinesiol.* **1999**, *9*, 385–389. [CrossRef] [PubMed]
22. Pohl, M.B.; Messenger, N.; Buckley, J.G. Changes in foot and lower limb coupling due to systematic variations in step width. *Clin. Biomech.* **2006**, *21*, 175–183. [CrossRef]
23. Eerdekens, M.; Peerlinck, K.; Staes, F.; Pialat, J.B.; Hermans, C.; Lobet, S.; Scheys, L.; Deschamps, K. Blood-induced cartilage damage alters the ankle joint load during walking. *J. Orthop. Res.* **2020**, *38*, 2419–2428. [CrossRef]
24. Bruening, D.A.; Pohl, M.B.; Takahashi, K.Z.; Barrios, J.A. Midtarsal locking, the windlass mechanism, and running strike pattern: A kinematic and kinetic assessment. *J. Biomech.* **2018**, *73*, 185–191. [CrossRef] [PubMed]
25. Hofbauer, M.; Thorhauer, E.D.; Abebe, E.; Bey, M.; Tashman, S. Altered tibiofemoral kinematics in the affected knee and compensatory changes in the contralateral knee after anterior cruciate ligament reconstruction. *Am. J. Sport. Med.* **2014**, *42*, 2715–2721. [CrossRef] [PubMed]
26. Smeeing DP, J.; Houwert, R.M.; Briet, J.P.; Kelder, J.C.; Segers MJ, M.; Verleisdonk EJ, M.M.; Leenen LP, H.; Hietbrink, F. Weight-bearing and mobilization in the postoperative care of ankle fractures: A systematic review and meta-analysis of randomized controlled trials and cohort studies. *PLoS ONE* **2015**, *10*, e0118320. [CrossRef] [PubMed]
27. Dehghan, N.; McKee, M.D.; Jenkinson, R.J.; Schemitsch, E.H.; Stas, V.; Nauth, A.; Hall, J.A.; Stephen, D.J.; Kreder, H.J. Early weightbearing and range of motion versus non-weightbearing and immobilization after open reduction and internal fixation of unstable ankle fractures: A randomized controlled trial. *J. Orthop. Trauma* **2016**, *30*, 345–352. [CrossRef]
28. Passias, B.J.; Korpi, F.P.; Chu, A.K.; Myers, D.M.; Grenier, G.; Galos, D.K.; Taylor, B. Safety of Early Weight Bearing Following Fixation of Bimalleolar Ankle Fractures. *Cureus* **2020**, *12*, e7557. [CrossRef] [PubMed]
29. Franklin, S.; Grey, M.J.; Heneghan, N.; Bowen, L.; Li, F.X. Barefoot vs common footwear: A systematic review of the kinematic, kinetic and muscle activity differences during walking. *Gait Posture* **2015**, *42*, 230–239. [CrossRef] [PubMed]

Disclaimer/Publisher's Note: The statements, opinions and data contained in all publications are solely those of the individual author(s) and contributor(s) and not of MDPI and/or the editor(s). MDPI and/or the editor(s) disclaim responsibility for any injury to people or property resulting from any ideas, methods, instructions or products referred to in the content.

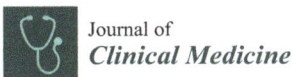

Article

Application of an Intraoperative Limb Positioner for Adjustable Traction in Both-Column Fractures of the Acetabulum: A Technical Note with Clinical Outcome

Joon-Woo Kim [1], Chang-Wug Oh [1,*], Kyeong-Hyeon Park [1], Won-Ki Hong [1], Sung-Hyuk Yoon [1], Gwang-Sub Lee [1] and Jong-Keon Oh [2]

1 Department of Orthopedic Surgery, School of Medicine, Kyungpook National University, Kyungpook National University Hospital, Jung-gu, Daegu 41944, Republic of Korea
2 Department of Orthopedic Surgery, School of Medicine, Korea University Guro Hospital, Seoul 10408, Republic of Korea
* Correspondence: cwoh@knu.ac.kr; Tel.: +82-53-420-5630

Abstract: Traction of the ipsilateral leg is usually required to facilitate fracture reduction while operating both-column acetabular fractures. However, it is challenging to maintain constant traction manually during the operation. Herein, we surgically treated such injuries while maintaining traction using an intraoperative limb positioner and investigated the outcomes. This study included 19 patients with both-column acetabular fractures. Surgery was performed after the patient's condition had stabilized, at an average of 10.4 days after injury. The Steinmann pin was transfixed to the distal femur and connected to a traction stirrup; subsequently, the construct was affixed to the limb positioner. A manual traction force was applied through the stirrup and maintained with the limb positioner. Using a modified Stoppa approach combined with the lateral window of the ilioinguinal approach, the fracture was reduced, and plates were applied. Primary union was achieved in all cases at an average of 17.3 weeks. The quality of reduction at the final follow-up was found to be excellent, good, and poor in 10, 8, and 1 patients, respectively. The average Merle d'Aubigné score at the final follow-up was 16.6. Surgical treatment of both-column acetabular fracture using intraoperative traction with a limb positioner yields satisfactory radiological and clinical outcomes.

Keywords: acetabular fracture; both-column fracture; intraoperative traction; limb positioner

Citation: Kim, J.-W.; Oh, C.-W.; Park, K.-H.; Hong, W.-K.; Yoon, S.-H.; Lee, G.-S.; Oh, J.-K. Application of an Intraoperative Limb Positioner for Adjustable Traction in Both-Column Fractures of the Acetabulum: A Technical Note with Clinical Outcome. *J. Clin. Med.* **2023**, *12*, 1682. https://doi.org/10.3390/jcm12041682

Academic Editors: Paul Alfred Grützner and Piettro Regazzoni

Received: 10 January 2023
Revised: 1 February 2023
Accepted: 17 February 2023
Published: 20 February 2023

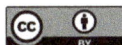

Copyright: © 2023 by the authors. Licensee MDPI, Basel, Switzerland. This article is an open access article distributed under the terms and conditions of the Creative Commons Attribution (CC BY) license (https://creativecommons.org/licenses/by/4.0/).

1. Introduction

Both-column fracture of the acetabulum is relatively common among acetabular fractures and is mainly caused by high-energy trauma [1,2]. During open reduction and internal fixation, intraoperative traction of the ipsilateral leg is required in most cases to facilitate fracture reduction and stabilization. In particular, in acetabular fractures associated with central dislocation of the femoral head, adequate reduction in the fracture is challenging without traction. Methods for applying intraoperative traction in pelvic and acetabular surgery are as follows: taking help from a skilled assistant for manual traction, using a universal distractor or external fixator, and using an on-table frame [3–6]; however, there is no consensus on an ideal technique [7]. In general, intraoperative traction is entirely dependent on surgical assistants because it is the simplest and most easily reproducible method, requiring no special equipment. However, it is not easy for humans to perform precise and continuous traction with constant force throughout the operation. Moreover, the surgical assistant can easily be exhausted, and the need for extra operating room personnel is another drawback.

Limb positioners, which were originally designed for upper extremity surgery and arthroscopic procedures, have been increasingly used in lower extremity procedures because they can be easily adjusted intraoperatively [8]. We hypothesized that both-column fractures of the acetabulum can also be effectively managed with intraoperative traction using a limb positioner. Accordingly, we describe our technique, which—to the best of our knowledge—has not yet been reported in patients with both-column fractures of the acetabulum. This study aimed to report on the novel use of a limb positioner as an intraoperative reduction aid for both-column fractures of the acetabulum as well as its clinical outcomes.

2. Materials and Methods

Our study included 19 patients, including 10 men and 9 women (mean age, 54 [range, 21–89] years) with both-column fractures of the acetabulum. Notably, the causes of the injury were traffic accidents and fall from a height in 13 and 6 patients, respectively. Of the 19 patients, 11 (57.8%) had a central dislocation of the femoral head. The average follow-up period was 30.5 (range, 12–60) months (Table 1). All surgeries were performed by two experienced surgeons (J.-W.K. and C.-W.O.), and the surgical team usually consisted of one surgeon and two assistants, sometimes one surgeon and one assistant.

Table 1. Patient's background and summarized results.

No.	Age	Sex	Injury Mechanism	Side	CDFH	Operation Time (Minutes)	Reduction Status (by Matta)	Union Time (Months)	Follow-Up Duration (Months)	Merle d'Aubigné Score	Complication
1	35	M	Driver accident	L	Yes	150	Excellent	16	40	15	
2	66	M	Pedestrian accident	R	Yes	240	Excellent	18	50	18	
3	89	F	Fall down	L	No	200	Good	17	30	18	
4	85	M	Motorcycle accident	R	Yes	180	Good	18	12	15	
5	60	F	Pedestrian accident	R	No	240	Excellent	16	32	15	
6	50	F	Pedestrian accident	R	No	190	Excellent	20	19	18	
7	55	M	Pedestrian accident	R	Yes	200	Good	20	60	15	
8	47	M	Pedestrian accident	L	Yes	250	Excellent	18	49	16	
9	21	F	Motorcycle accident	R	Yes	240	Excellent	15	29	15	
10	55	M	Fall down	L	No	180	Good	20	30	17	
11	58	M	Fall down	L	No	220	Excellent	18	24	16	
12	56	M	Pedestrian accident	R	Yes	240	Good	18	28	16	
13	71	F	Pedestrian accident	R	No	200	Good	16	23	15	ONFH
14	50	M	Fall down	R	Yes	155	Excellent	16	23	18	
15	25	F	Fall down	R	Yes	180	Excellent	18	30	18	
16	60	F	Driver accident	L	No	170	Good	18	26	18	
17	31	M	Fall down	R	Yes	240	Excellent	16	34	18	
18	64	F	Pedestrian accident	R	Yes	290	Poor	18	17	15	
19	44	F	Pedestrian accident	R	No	200	Good	13	24	18	Traumatic OA

M: male, F: female, CDFH: Central dislocation of the femoral head, ONFH: Osteonecrosis of the femoral head, OA: osteoarthritis.

2.1. Operative Technique

1. Preparation

After the induction of general anesthesia, the patient was placed in a supine position on a radiolucent table. The patient's both arms were placed on the arm board at 90° abduction. A shoulder support was placed on both axillae with a jelly pad to prevent the patient from getting pulled down while maintaining longitudinal traction with a limb positioner (Figure 1). Further, an image intensifier was introduced from the contralateral side.

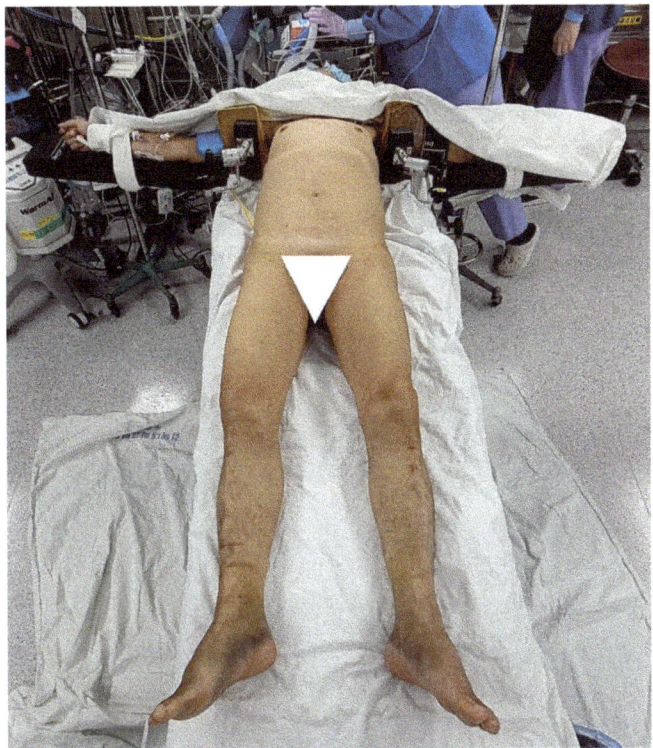

Figure 1. After anesthesia, the patient was placed in a supine position with both arms abducted at 90°. A shoulder support was placed on both axillae with a jelly pad to prevent the patient from getting pulled down while maintaining longitudinal traction with a limb positioner.

The entire ipsilateral lower limb was then prepared and freely draped to facilitate the intraoperative reduction maneuver. Notably, sterile draping was extended proximally to the subcostal region. A pillow was placed underneath the popliteal fossa for slight flexion of the hip in order to relax the iliopsoas muscle.

2. Traction with a limb positioner

To insert a pin for traction, the knee was flexed to 30° with neutral rotation. Using a pointed scalpel, a stab incision was made through the skin on the medial side 2–3 finger breadths above the superior pole of the patella. After placing a 3.2 mm Steinmann pin on the drill, insertion was made parallel to the joint line from the medial to lateral sides. Further, after driving the Steinmann pin through the bone and ensuring that the pin had penetrated the far cortex, another stab incision was made on the overlying skin, coinciding with the expected exit of the pin. After the Steinmann pin was completely out, the tension on the skin at the entry and exit points was checked. A small relieving incision was additionally performed in case of excessive tension.

The Steinmann pin was transfixed and then connected with a traction stirrup and affixed to the limb positioner (The Spider Limb Positioner, Smith and Nephew®, Andover, MA, USA). Sterility was assured by first covering the limb positioner with the manufacturer's sterile drape and then proceeding with standard sterile pelvic draping (Figure 2). Subsequently, sufficient manual traction force was applied through the stirrup, and the degree of reduction was confirmed using an image intensifier (Figure 3). The stirrup was then connected to the pneumatic limb positioner and locked while maintaining traction (Figure 2D and Video S1).

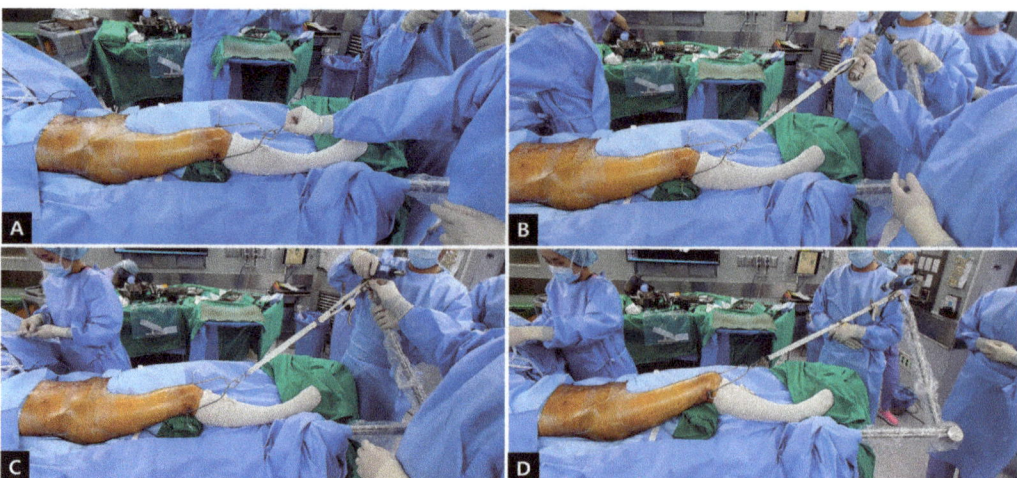

Figure 2. After transfixing the Steinmann pin in the distal femur, it was connected with a traction stirrup (**A**). The Stein-mann pin-traction stirrup construct was affixed to the limb positioner (**B**). Sufficient manual traction force was applied through the stirrup (**C**). The limb positioner was locked while maintaining traction (**D**).

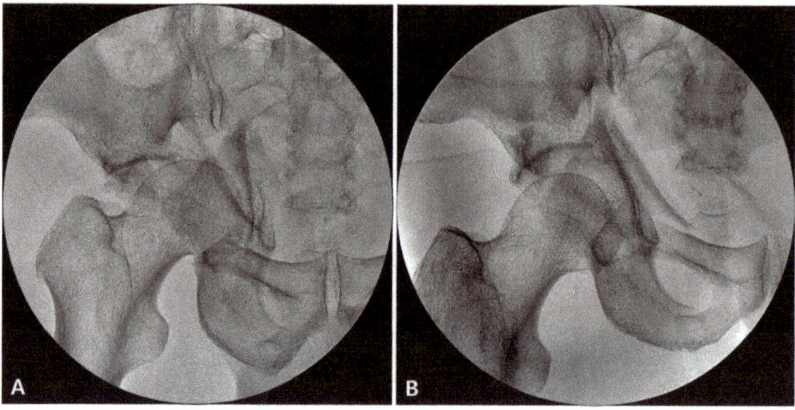

Figure 3. Intraoperative image before (**A**) and after (**B**) traction.

3. Reduction and fixation

We used a modified Stoppa approach combined with a lateral window of the ilioinguinal approach. First, we aimed to reduce the displaced anterior column to the posterior ilium. A 5.0 mm Schanz screw was inserted in the anterior inferior iliac spine, and the iliac wing was internally rotated. The elevated anterior column fragment was squeezed out using a ball spike pusher. A 5–6-hole reconstruction plate or small locking compression plate was undercontoured and placed at the junction of the fracture line along the pelvic brim. The distal part of the plate was placed on the free anterior column fragment, and cortical screws were fixed to the proximal portion of the plate—the stable portion of the posterior ilium. With the tightening of the screws, the under-bent plate pressed the anterior column fragment into alignment with the intact ilium. Cortical screws were then fixed into the distal portion of the plate while exercising caution to avoid pulling the anterior column fragment. We also performed reduction and fixation of the iliac wing with a lag screw or reconstruction plate, if required.

Subsequently, the posterior column was reduced. Notably, as this column was already almost reduced by ligamentotaxis via traction through the limb positioner in most cases, only fine adjustment or augmentation was required. The pelvic arm of the collinear reduction clamp was placed in the lesser sciatic notch from the lateral window of the ilioinguinal approach. Further, the collinear reduction clamp was assembled with the pelvic arm and gently squeezed while observing the reduction status via the Stoppa window. After confirming that the quadrilateral surface was adequately reduced to the anterior column via direct visualization, a 3.5 mm long lag screw was placed in the direction of the ischial spine. We made it a rule to place at least two screws for the posterior column fixation.

Finally, a curved 12-hole pelvic reconstruction plate was contoured and applied along the pelvic brim, from the innominate bone adjacent to the sacroiliac joint to the pubic tubercle. Remarkably, the plate was introduced from the lateral window of the ilioinguinal approach in the direction of the distal Stoppa incision. The cranial- and caudal-most screws were placed to buttress and stabilize the reduced anterior column fragment. An additional posterior column screw was placed through the plate hole or separately next to the plate hole if required.

The fixation status was confirmed using an intraoperative image intensifier in the anteroposterior, iliac wing, and obturator oblique views. If a large posterior wall fragment was present or the posterior column reduction was unsatisfactory, they were corrected and stabilized using a separate posterior approach. After completion of all fixations, the traction was released and a final radiographic assessment was performed before wound closure.

2.2. Postoperative Management and Assessment

Patients were encouraged to sit up within the first 24–48 h after surgery, and active hip and knee joint motions were advised. Partial weight bearing was allowed with crutches for 8 weeks after the operation, and this progressively increased to full weight bearing after 8 weeks. Further, sequential follow-up radiographs of the anteroposterior, iliac wing, and obturator oblique views of the pelvis were obtained at regular intervals of 4–8 weeks.

In radiological evaluations, healing rate, time to union, quality of reduction, and complications were assessed. Based on these findings, the quality of reduction was graded as excellent, good, fair, and poor according to Matta's criteria [9]. Moreover, the clinical results were graded as excellent, good, fair, and poor according to the modified Merle d'Aubigné scoring system (excellent, 18; good, 15–17; fair, 12–14; poor, <12), which is based on the assessments of pain, walking, and range of motion.

3. Results

Operative fixation was performed at an average of 10.4 (range, 4–22) days after patients were appropriately resuscitated and optimized for surgery. Seven patients had multiple fractures, including spine, forearm, tibial, and ankle fractures. Two patients sustained various chest traumas, such as flail chest, pneumo-/hemothorax, and multiple rib fractures. Two patients sustained a liver injury that required emergency intervention.

Overall, 16 of the 19 patients underwent surgery via the anterior approach alone, whereas three patients required additional posterior fixation through a separate posterior approach. The mean operation time was 208.6 min (range, 150–290). Primary bone union was achieved in all cases at an average of 17.3 (range, 15–20) weeks. The quality of reduction assessed by Matta's criteria at the final follow-up was excellent, good, and poor in 10, 8, and 1 patients, respectively. Notably, all patients achieved excellent or good functional outcomes with a median Merle d'Aubigné score of 16.6 (range, 15–18), except for two patients.

These two patients (10.5%) underwent hip arthroplasty at 5 and 11 months postoperatively, respectively. One patient had a severe femoral head impaction at the time of injury, and osteonecrosis of the femoral head, followed by secondary arthritis, was found to be rapidly progressing. The other patient sustained severe comminution of the acetabular cartilage. Although the postoperative reduction status was relatively satisfactory, joint space narrowing gradually progressed and osteoarthritis eventually developed with complaints of severe pain.

Complications caused by continuous traction, such as nerve or vascular damage, pin site problems, or pressure sore, were not observed in any case.

4. Discussion

Reduction is the first and most important step in acetabular surgery. Intraoperative traction is essential to neutralize the deforming force that caused the fracture, and it facilitates the reduction. Various intraoperative traction methods have been described in the relevant literature, including the use of a surgical assistant to provide intermittent manual traction, an external fixator, a fracture table, or an on-table frame [7]. A skilled assistant can apply manual traction, but the assistant can easily be exhausted, and the need for additional operating room personnel is another drawback. Moreover, a previous study reported that the major disadvantage of using a radiolucent table is the need for manual traction; thus, it requires a minimum of two or three assistants [10]. In addition, it is difficult for a human to apply a constant force throughout the operation. In contrast, the benefit of using the fracture table is that constant and precise traction can be maintained indefinitely, although an additional surgical assistant is still required to operate the table. However, the design of the fracture table limits certain movements of the extremity and interferes with certain fluoroscopic views [11–13]. Notably, an on-table frame can be used for this purpose, but force vectors are two-dimensional [5]. Moreover, external fixators or distractors can be used, although traction is most commonly provided along a single defined vector in these techniques [3–6]. In contrast, the method described in our study does not require additional personnel, and the number of assistants can be decreased. Before using limb positioner traction, our surgical team for a pelvic-acetabular fracture usually consisted of one surgeon and three assistants, whereas two assistants are sufficient after using this method. In addition, it is easily adjustable and can be manipulated in multiple vectors simultaneously. An additional advantage is that the distraction direction, which facilitates fracture reduction, can be adjusted and maintained and, if necessary, easily changed during the operation. Similarly, compared with other table attachments that offer only leg movement, a particular advantage of the limb positioner is that the leg can be manipulated in rotation and flexion/extension while engaged [7]. In addition to having complete freedom of leg position when initially applying traction, it is easy to adjust it as often as preferred. Furthermore, since most centers performing limb surgery are generally furnished with a limb positioner, it is also considered to be cost effective to use this as a traction device in this respect.

The Spider Limb Positioner is a pneumatic arm with three fully articulated joints that uses compressed air or nitrogen to facilitate its static locking mechanisms. It was classically used for shoulder arthroscopic procedures. The foot pedal allows the surgeon to control the limb during surgery and is the means by which pressurized air or nitrogen is supplied to the pneumatic arm. Notably, the foot pedal unlocks the three joints simultaneously, allowing the repositioning of the limb in an infinite number of positions while maintaining a sterile field [8]. Additionally, the limb can be connected to and disconnected from the limb positioner while maintaining a sterile field throughout the procedure. Owing to the limb positioner's unique ability to allow infinite positional adjustments in three dimensions, we aimed to use it for intraoperative traction. Furthermore, the limb positioner can support a maximum of 22.3 kg (50 lbs) [8], which is believed to provide sufficient strength for traction.

In a previous study of both-column acetabular fracture, the hip joint was congruent in 94.7% after surgery, which is comparable to our result [2]. However, they experienced 8.9% of iatrogenic nerve injuries and 60.7% of patients had the mean Merle d'Aubigné score of 15, and 25.8% of the patients diagnosed a joint failure, which is somewhat inferior to ours. The operation time in the current study was also relatively shorter than described in previous studies [2,14,15]. It is believed that this is because the operation can be performed while maintaining stable traction with the limb positioner, without repetitive actions for reduction.

To the best of our knowledge, no case series has described the use of a limb positioner as a reduction tool with clinical and radiological outcomes in both-column fractures of the acetabulum with adequate follow-up, although a previous case report described the technique of lateral traction for reduction of the medialized femoral head using a limb positioner [7]. Although intraoperative traction using a limb positioner may not have a significant effect on the clinical and radiological outcome, it is considered to be true that the surgical procedure can be convenient and efficient.

This study has some limitations. First, the study used a retrospective design and a small cohort size. Second, the unconventional use of a limb positioner for traction purposes is not authorized. However, considering that this is a novel attempt to introduce the limb positioner in acetabular fracture surgery, we believe that it deserves attention as it can provide acetabular surgeons with a new reliable traction technique. In addition, this can be a reasonable and safe alternative technique to maintain intraoperative traction when operating both-column fractures of the acetabulum.

5. Conclusions

Surgical treatment of both-column fractures of the acetabulum using intraoperative adjustable traction with a limb positioner is considered an effective and safe method because it allows continuous traction with constant force throughout the surgery and without any traction-related complications. It also helps to reduce and stabilize the fracture, reduces the number of required operating room personnel, and yields favorable radiologic and functional outcomes.

Supplementary Materials: The following supporting information can be downloaded at: https://www.mdpi.com/article/10.3390/jcm12041682/s1, Table S1: Patient's background and summarized results; Video S1: The process of applying the limb positioner for intraoperative traction.

Author Contributions: Conceptualization, J.-W.K. and C.-W.O.; methodology, K.-H.P. and W.-K.H.; validation, J.-W.K. and W.-K.H.; formal analysis, S.-H.Y. and G.-S.L.; investigation, K.-H.P. and S.-H.Y.; data curation, J.-W.K. and G.-S.L.; writing—original draft preparation, J.-W.K.; writing—review and editing, C.-W.O.; visualization, J.-K.O.; supervision, C.-W.O. All authors have read and agreed to the published version of the manuscript.

Funding: This research was supported by a grant of the Korea Health Technology R&D Project through the Korea Health Industry Development Institute (KHIDI), funded by the Ministry of Health & Welfare, Republic of Korea (grant number: HR22C1832).

Institutional Review Board Statement: The study design and protocol were approved by the institutional review board of Kyungpook National University Hospital (IRB No.: 2021-04-025).

Informed Consent Statement: Informed consent was obtained from all subjects involved in the study.

Data Availability Statement: Source data may be shared upon reasonable request to the corresponding author.

Conflicts of Interest: The authors declare no conflict of interest.

References

1. Kelly, J.; Ladurner, A.; Rickman, M. Surgical management of acetabular fractures—A contemporary literature review. *Injury* **2020**, *51*, 2267–2271. [CrossRef] [PubMed]
2. Gänsslen, A.; Frink, M.; Hildebrand, F.; Krettek, C. Both column fractures of the acetabulum: Epidemiology, operative management and long-term-results. *Acta Chir. Orthop. Traumatol. Cech.* **2012**, *79*, 107–113. [PubMed]
3. Tannast, M.; Najibi, S.; Matta, J.M. Two to twenty-year survivorship of the hip in 810 patients with operatively treated acetabular fractures. *J. Bone Jt. Surg. Am.* **2012**, *94*, 1559–1567. [CrossRef] [PubMed]
4. Calafi, L.A.; Routt, M.L. Direct hip joint distraction during acetabular fracture surgery using the AO universal manipulator. *J. Trauma Inj. Infect. Crit. Care* **2010**, *68*, 481–484. [CrossRef] [PubMed]
5. Lefaivre, K.A.; Starr, A.J.; Barker, B.P.; Overturf, S.; Reinert, C.M. Early experience with reduction of displaced disruption of the pelvic ring using a pelvic reduction frame. *J. Bone Jt. Surg. Br.* **2009**, *91*, 1201–1207. [CrossRef]

6. Romanelli, F.; Boe, E.; Sun, L.; Keller, D.M.; Yoon, R.S.; Liporace, F.A. Temporary external fixation to table as a traction reduction aide in the treatment of unstable pelvic ring injuries: A technical note. *Hip Pelvis* **2020**, *32*, 214–222. [CrossRef]
7. Goodnough, L.H.; Olsen, T.; Hidden, K.; DeBaun, M.R.; Kleweno, C.P. Use of an intraoperative limb positioner for adjustable distraction in acetabulum fractures with femoral head protrusion: A case report. *JBJS Case Connect.* **2021**, *8*, 11. [CrossRef] [PubMed]
8. Henderson, E.R.; Prioreschi, B.; Mata-Fink, A.; Bell, J.E. Use of the spider limb positioner in oncologic lower extremity surgery. *Expert Rev. Med. Devices* **2014**, *11*, 581–585. [CrossRef] [PubMed]
9. Matta, J. Fractures of the acetabulum: Accuracy of reduction and clinical results of fractures operated within three weeks after the injury. *J. Bone Jt. Surg. Am.* **1996**, *78*, 1632–1645. [CrossRef]
10. Rommens, P.M. Ilioinguinal approach for acetabular fractures. *Orthop. Traumatol.* **2002**, *10*, 179–189. [CrossRef]
11. Giannoudis, P.V.; Grotz, M.R.; Papakostidis, C.; Dinopoulos, H. Operative treatment of displaced fractures of the acetabulum. A meta-analysis. *J. Bone Jt. Surg. Br.* **2005**, *87*, 2–9. [CrossRef]
12. Tile, M.; Helfet, D.; Kellam, J. *Fractures of the Pelvis and the Acetabulum*, 3rd ed.; Lippincott Williams & Wilkins: New York, NY, USA, 2003.
13. Harris, A.M.; Althausen, P.; Kellam, J.F.; Bosse, M.J. Simultaneous anterior and posterior approaches for complex acetabular fractures. *J. Orthop. Trauma* **2008**, *22*, 494–497. [CrossRef] [PubMed]
14. Chen, C.; Chiu, E.; Lo, W.; Chung, T. Cerclage wiring in displaced both column fractures of the acetabulum. *Injury* **2001**, *32*, 391–394. [CrossRef] [PubMed]
15. Masahiro, S.; Kensei, N.; Kensuke, S.; Kunihiko, T.; Takanobu, A.; Toshiya, E.; Kmanabu, K.; Masabumi, I.; Toyama, U. Operative treatment of both column fractures in the acetabulum. *Orthop. Traumatol.* **2002**, *51*, 162–167.

Disclaimer/Publisher's Note: The statements, opinions and data contained in all publications are solely those of the individual author(s) and contributor(s) and not of MDPI and/or the editor(s). MDPI and/or the editor(s) disclaim responsibility for any injury to people or property resulting from any ideas, methods, instructions or products referred to in the content.

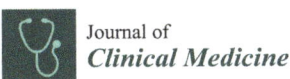

Article

Minimally Invasive Derotational Osteotomy of Long Bones: Smartphone Application Used to Improve the Accuracy of Correction

Chang-Wug Oh [1], Kyeong-Hyeon Park [2,*], Joon-Woo Kim [1], Dong-Hyun Kim [1], Il Seo [1], Jin-Han Lee [1], Ji-Wan Kim [3] and Sung-Hyuk Yoon [1]

[1] Department of Orthopedic Surgery, School of Medicine, Kyungpook National University, Kyungpook National University Hospital, Daegu 41944, Republic of Korea
[2] Department of Orthopedic Surgery, Severance Children's Hospital, Yonsei University College of Medicine, Seoul 03722, Republic of Korea
[3] Department of Orthopedic Surgery, Asan Medical Center, University of Ulsan College of Medicine, Seoul 05505, Republic of Korea
* Correspondence: pkh1112@gmail.com; Tel.: +82-53-420-5628

Abstract: Correction of rotational malalignments caused by fractures is essential as it may cause pain and gait disturbances. This study evaluated the intraoperative use of a smartphone application (SP app) to measure the extent of corrective rotation in patients treated using minimally invasive derotational osteotomy. Intraoperatively, two parallel 5 mm Schanz pins were placed above and below the fractured/injured site, and derotation was performed manually after percutaneous osteotomy. A protractor SP app was used intraoperatively to measure the angle between the two Schanz pins (angle-SP). Intramedullary nailing or minimally invasive plate osteosynthesis was performed after derotation, and computerized tomography (CT) scans were used to assess the angle of correction postoperatively (angle-CT). The accuracy of rotational correction was assessed by comparing angle-SP and angle-CT. The mean preoperative rotational difference observed was 22.1°, while the mean angle-SP and angle-CT were 21.6° and 21.3°, respectively. A significant positive correlation between angle-SP and angle-CT was observed, and 18 out of 19 patients exhibited complete healing within 17.7 weeks (1 patient exhibited nonunion). These findings suggest that using an SP app during minimally invasive derotational osteotomy can result in accurate correction of malrotation of long bones in a reproducible manner. Therefore, SP technology with integrated gyroscope function represents a suitable alternative for determination of the magnitude of rotational correction when performing corrective osteotomy.

Keywords: derotational osteotomy; malrotation; rotational malalignment; smartphone application

Citation: Oh, C.-W.; Park, K.-H.; Kim, J.-W.; Kim, D.-H.; Seo, I.; Lee, J.-H.; Kim, J.-W.; Yoon, S.-H. Minimally Invasive Derotational Osteotomy of Long Bones: Smartphone Application Used to Improve the Accuracy of Correction. *J. Clin. Med.* **2023**, *12*, 1335. https://doi.org/10.3390/jcm12041335

Academic Editors: Umile Giuseppe Longo and Pengde Kang

Received: 29 December 2022
Revised: 22 January 2023
Accepted: 6 February 2023
Published: 7 February 2023

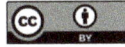

Copyright: © 2023 by the authors. Licensee MDPI, Basel, Switzerland. This article is an open access article distributed under the terms and conditions of the Creative Commons Attribution (CC BY) license (https://creativecommons.org/licenses/by/4.0/).

1. Introduction

Intramedullary (IM) nailing and minimally invasive plate osteosynthesis (MIPO) are the most commonly used treatment measures for diaphyseal and metaphyseal fractures of long bones, respectively [1,2]. These closed-reduction surgical techniques provide better treatment outcomes (e.g., excellent fracture healing and rapid patient recovery) compared to open reduction with internal fixation, as they require smaller incisions and minimal soft tissue dissection. Malrotation, a common complication of IM nailing or MIPO, is often overlooked in comparison to angular deformities of the coronal and sagittal planes. Postoperative malrotations exceeding 10° have been observed in 50% of patients with femoral and tibial fractures [3–6], and restoration of the alignment is essential as abnormal loading may lead to pain, instability, and early degeneration [7].

Although challenging, a variety of osteotomy procedures have been used previously for the correction of rotational malalignment. During open osteotomy, the surgeon marks reference lines over the bone and/or uses angle templates to visually determine the desired correction intraoperatively [8]. This traditional technique can disturb bone healing and increase blood loss through extensile exposure, and this risk can be decreased by using minimally invasive corrective osteotomy techniques with fluoroscopic guidance [9,10]. Although intraoperative C-arm images have been used for objective measurement of the lesser trochanter profile, cortical step sign, and diameter difference sign [11,12], visual fluoroscopic estimation may prove to be imprecise when determining the angle of rotation [13].

Although the gyroscopic function of smartphone (SP) technology has previously been used to measure angles in bone models simulating rotational deformities [14,15], there is limited evidence of its efficacy in measuring the rotational angle during surgical corrective osteotomy. Therefore, in the current study, a consecutive series of derotational osteotomies were performed using an SP application (SP app) intraoperatively, and a comparison of the desired angle, measured using the SP app, and the corrected angle, measured using a postoperative CT scan, was carried out. The hypothesis being tested was that the proposed osteotomy technique using an SP app would achieve accurate correction of rotational deformity in a reproducible manner.

2. Materials and Methods

This study was approved by the ethics committee of the institute, and informed consent was collected from all participants prior to commencement of this study and after provision of relevant verbal and written information. Patients diagnosed with malunion/nonunion and rotational malalignment secondary to surgical intervention for femoral or tibial fractures were selected to undergo the proposed procedure. A thorough evaluation of the diagnosis was carried out to identify any additional requirements during the surgical procedure.

The indication is based on symptoms and clinical and radiological evaluation. No clear indications for surgical correction are reported in the literature. Patients were included if they met any of the following criteria:

1. Malrotation of more than 15 degrees after fracture surgery;
2. Malrotation greater than 10 degrees in nonunion patients;
3. Among patients with malrotation of more than 15 degrees and symptomatic patellofemoral malalignment interfering with daily life.

Patients were excluded if the patient refused additional surgery or had asymptomatic malrotation.

In addition to standard radiographic evaluation, all patients underwent preoperative computerized tomography (CT) scans to allow accurate identification of anatomical deformities. Femoral torsion was determined by measuring the angle between the long axis of the femoral neck and a line drawn parallel to the dorsal aspect of the femoral condyles on an axial CT image [16] (Figure 1). Tibial torsion was defined as the angle between the posterior tibial axis of the proximal tibia and the bimalleolar axis of the distal tibia on an axial CT image [17]. The difference in the angle of rotational alignment of the affected and contralateral unaffected limbs was calculated.

2.1. Surgical Technique

Preoperative evaluation included calculation of the required angulation of rotational correction and identification of any additional deformities. The surgical plan included derotational osteotomy at the previously fractured area and use of either an IM nail or plate for fixation, selected based on the anatomical location of the pre-existing implant.

During surgery, the patient was placed in a supine or lateral position on a radiolucent table, and their whole lower extremity was draped. Prior to commencement of the osteotomy, two parallel 5 mm Schanz pins were carefully placed above and below the previous fracture such that they did not interfere with the pre-existing or new implants (nail or plate) to allow accurate measurement of the correction (Figure 2).

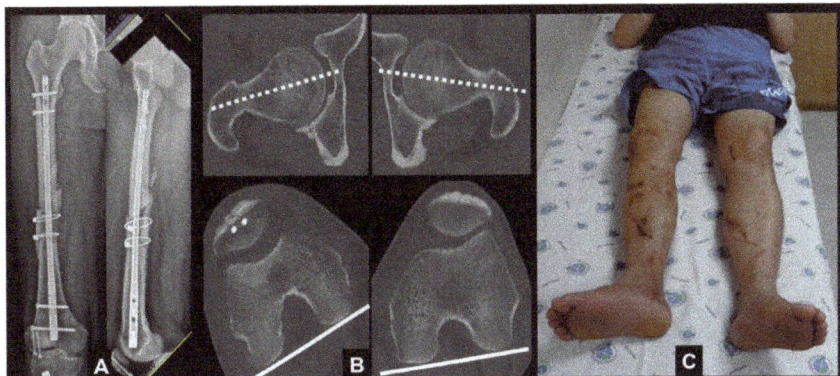

Figure 1. (**A**) Preoperative anteroposterior and lateral radiographs showing nonunion after retrograde nailing; (**B**) CT scan showing an evident difference in the femoral torsional angle between the affected and unaffected sides; (**C**) externally rotated foot on the right side indicating retroversion of the femur.

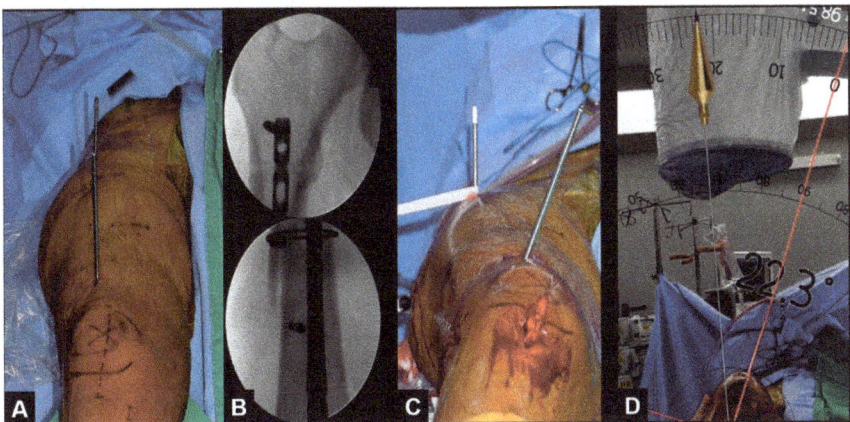

Figure 2. (**A**,**B**) Two parallel Schanz pins placed above and below the nonunion without interfering with the nail; (**C**) internal rotation of the distal segment after removal of the previous nail; (**D**) the smartphone application measured a 22° correction.

Thereafter, the pre-existing implant placed during the earlier osteosynthesis was removed, and in patients with nonunion or malunion, percutaneous osteotomy was performed at the planned site. Minimally invasive osteotomy was performed using a 1–2 cm incision and multiaxial drilling with C-arm control, and the final procedure was completed by connecting the multiple drill holes using a half-inch osteotome (Figure 3). In patients with postoperative malalignment, the proximal or distal fixation was disassembled without removing the full implant (Figures 4–9).

After reaming the medullary canal, a new IM nail was inserted, and derotation was carried out by manually rotating the distal part of the limb. The extent of rotation was estimated by measuring the angle between the two Schanz pins. The intraoperative angle of correction was measured by an assistant standing at the end of the table using a free protractor SP app (angle-SP). The corrective osteotomy aimed to achieve an angle of correction equivalent to the rotational alignment of the contralateral side, determined using a preoperative CT scan. A maximum difference of 5° between the measured and target values was considered acceptable. Distal fixation was then performed while maintaining the rotational correction, and the Schanz pins were removed. Clinical examination was performed after removal of the drapes to confirm rotational correction, and the patient was then sent to the recovery room.

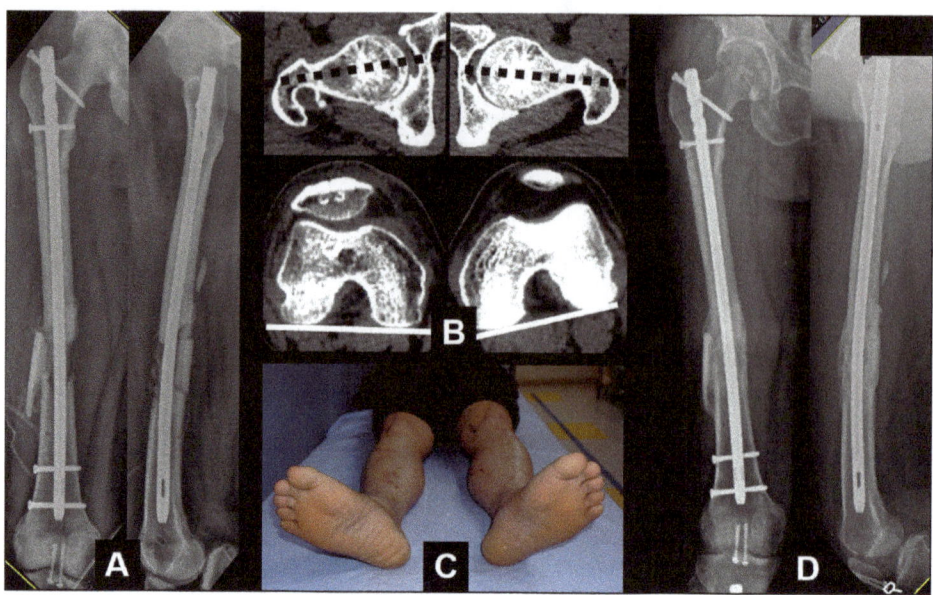

Figure 3. (**A**) Postoperative radiographs showing antegrade nailing with bone graft at the nonunion site; (**B**) CT scan showing similar angles of anteversion; (**C**) similar rotation in foot position; (**D**) complete healing observed 1 year postoperatively.

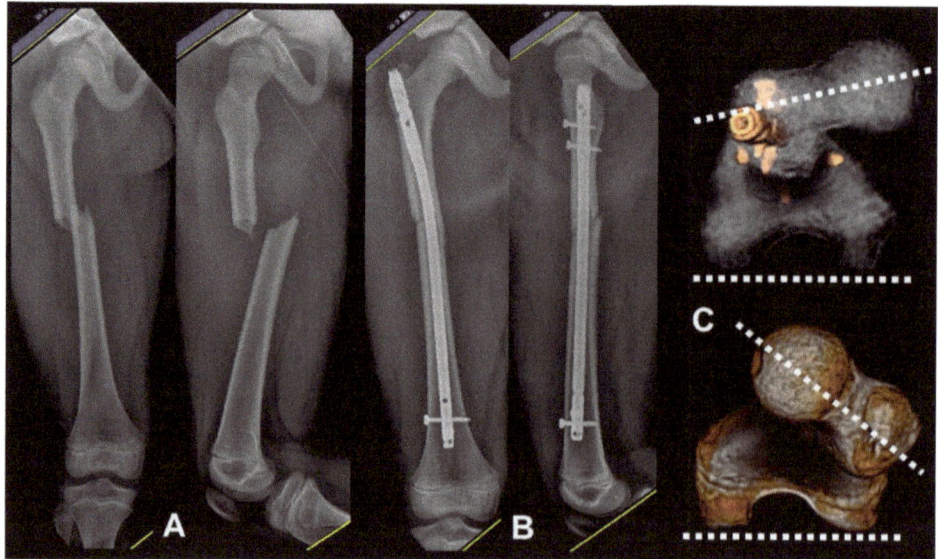

Figure 4. (**A**) An 11-year-old male patient diagnosed with a femoral-shaft fracture; (**B**) IM nailing was carried out; (**C**) postoperative CT scan showing the decreased angle of anteversion compared with the noninjured side.

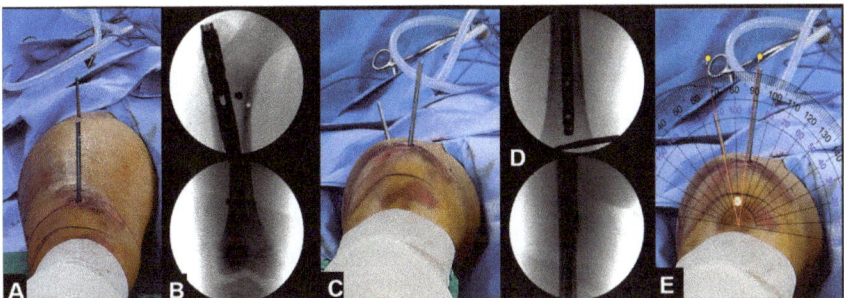

Figure 5. (**A**,**B**) Parallel Schanz pins placed in the proximal and distal femur; (**C**,**D**) internal rotation of the distal segment after removal of the distal interlocking screws; (**E**) the smartphone application measured a 20° correction.

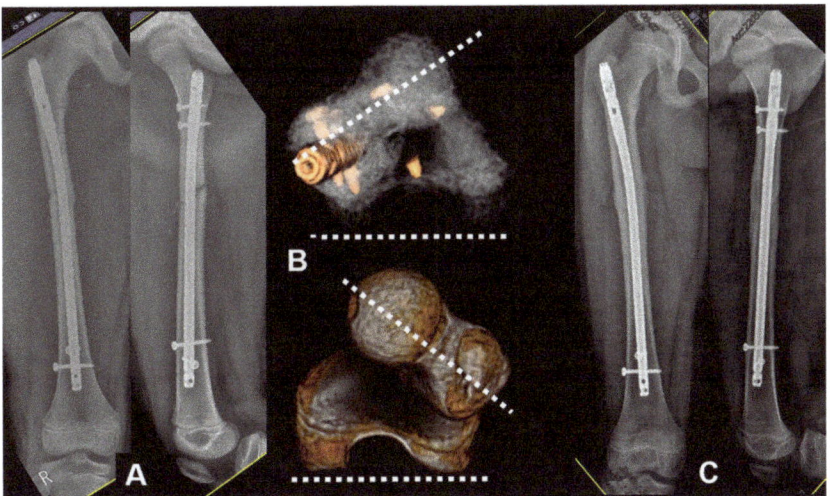

Figure 6. (**A**) Postoperative radiographs showing revised fixation of distal interlocking; (**B**) CT scan showing similar angles of anteversion; (**C**) complete healing observed 6 months postoperatively.

2.2. Smart Phone Application

The SP application (SP app) used in this study was the Smart Protractor application (Smart Tools Co., Dae-gu, South Korea). Measurement with the SP app is obtained by positioning a virtual protractor, visible on the SP screen, on photography obtained using the SP camera. The assistant takes a photo of the Schanz pins, saves it, measures the angles, and observes the value. The picture should be taken with the camera positioned along the imaginary line between two pins. After the photo has been taken and saved, two red lines appear on the screen. The lines can be dragged across the screen to place the virtual goniometer on the axis of the Schanz pins, finely adjusting them until the goniometer is positioned correctly. Pictures judged subjectively wrong by the surgeon because of a perspective error can be deleted. The angle-SP measurement was repeated three times, and the average value was determined.

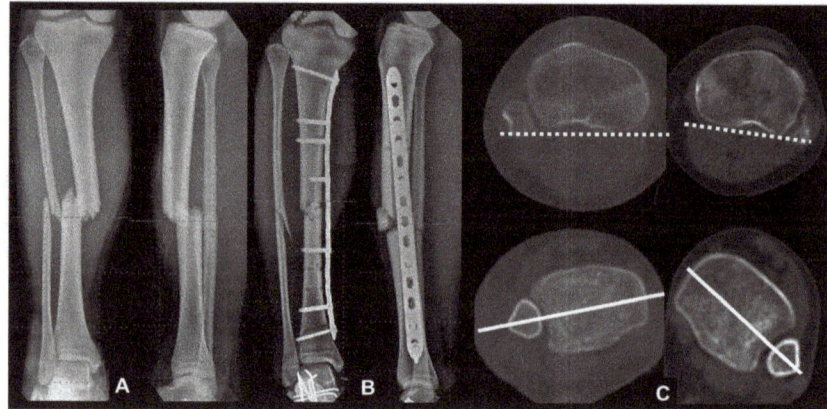

Figure 7. (**A**) A 15-year-old girl with a tibia shaft fracture; (**B**) minimally invasive plate osteosynthesis was carried out; (**C**) postoperative CT scan showing a moderate difference (over 16 degrees) in rotation compared with the noninjured side.

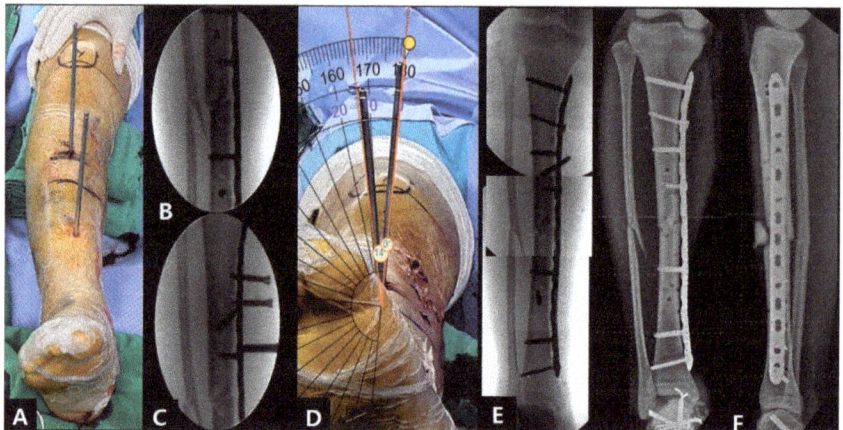

Figure 8. (**A**,**B**) Parallel Schanz pins placed in the proximal and distal tibia; (**C**) screws were removed at the proximal segment; (**D**) external rotation of the distal segment and the smartphone application measured about 14° correction; (**E**) screws were fixed at the proximal segment; (**F**) postoperative radiographs showing the improved alignment after revision procedure.

2.3. Postoperative Care and Evaluation

Postsurgical clinical evaluation of rotational correction involved comparison of foot rotation and internal and external rotation of the hip joint between the affected and unaffected limbs while the patient was still in the supine position on the table. Based on the patient's level of tolerance, range of motion was resumed slowly, and all patients were allowed use of partial weight-bearing crutches.

Postoperative CT scans were used to compare the angles (angle-CT), and a maximum difference of 5° was considered acceptable. The correlation between angle-SP (measured intraoperatively with the SP app) and angle-CT (measured postoperatively using a CT scan) was assessed.

Clinical follow-up was carried out 1, 2, and 3 months postoperatively, and every 3 months thereafter until bone union was achieved. Radiographic evaluation was carried out at each visit, and bone union was defined as the presence of an appropriate bridging callus and resolution of persistent fracture lines in at least 3 out of 4 radiographic views.

All patient radiographs were assessed by two independent board-certified orthopedic surgeons.

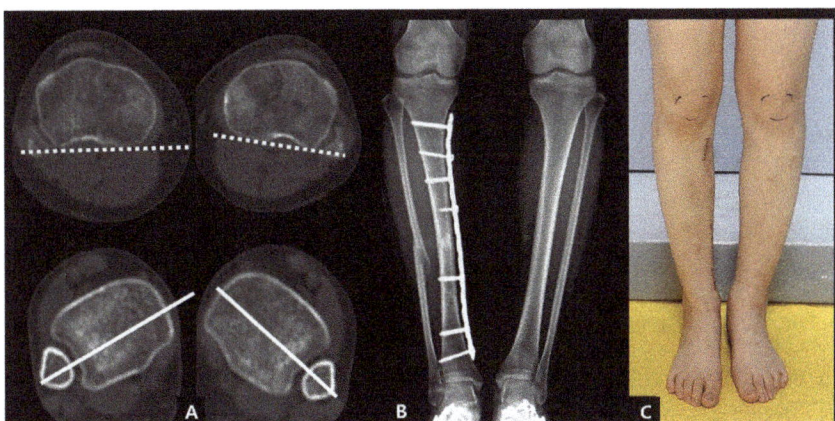

Figure 9. (**A**) Postoperative CT scan showing similar angles of rotation; (**B,C**) complete healing with the similar alignment of lower leg was observed 1 year postoperatively.

2.4. Statistical Analysis

Paired *t*-test and Pearson's correlation coefficient tests were used to compare the angle-SP and angle-CT, and all statistical analyses were performed using the IBM SPSS software, version 19.0 (IBM Co., Armonk, NY, USA). A *p*-value < 0.05 was considered statistically significant.

3. Results

Between March 2013 and February 2021, of the 31 identified patients who underwent derotational osteotomy in the femur or tibia, 19 patients treated with minimally invasive osteotomy with the SP app were included. Among 19 cases (17 cases of the femur, 2 cases of the tibia), 17 cases were treated using IM nailing, and 2 cases using MIPO. All patients had a minimum follow-up of 1 year. The mean age of the patients at the time of surgery was 37.9 years (range: 11–77 years).

Four patients were diagnosed with acute postoperative malalignment, 15 patients with late manifestation (nonunion $n = 12$; malunion, $n = 3$), 11 patients with externally rotated deformities, and 8 patients with internally rotated deformities. Preoperative CT scans showed a mean difference of 22.3° (range: 11.2°–38.3°) in rotational angle. Among those exhibiting nonunion, four patients presented with additional angular malalignments that were simultaneously corrected. Fixation was carried out using IM and MIPO in 17 and 2 patients, respectively, and additional bone grafting was carried out in 8 patients. Sixteen patients were operated on in the supine position, while three were in the lateral position.

The mean intraoperative angle-SP was 21.6° (range: 10.2°–36.1°), while the postoperative angle-CT was 21.3° (range: 13.9°–39.2°). The mean difference in angle of rotation was 2.3°, and the variations in value were within the accepted range of 5° (range: −4.2° to +4.8°). A statistically significant positive correlation between angle-SP and angle-CT was observed (Pearson's correlation coefficient $r = 0.972$; *p*-value = <0.001).

The mean duration of healing was 17.7 weeks (range: 12–24 weeks) in 18 out of 19 patients, and all of them exhibited acceptable improvement in gait with symmetric angles of foot progression. One patient exhibited nonunion requiring a secondary bone graft, while three patients presented with minor complications related to the Schanz pins (bent pin $n = 2$; broken pin, $n = 1$), which likely occurred during manual derotational correction. None of the patients developed any infections (Table 1).

Table 1. Patient demographics and outcomes.

No.	Sex	Age (Year)	Location	Cause	Rotational Deformity	Associated Deformity	Implant	Bone Graft	Pre-Operative Difference	Angle Measured Using SP App	Post-Operative Difference	Gained Angle	Time to Union (Weeks)
1	M	15	Femur	Malalignment	Internal		Nail	none	16.1	15.8	2.3	13.8	12
2	M	37	Femur	Nonunion	External		Nail	YES	38.3	36.1	3.2	35.1	16
3	M	22	Femur	Malalignment	External		Nail	none	22.3	20.9	-1.5	23.8	16
4	M	49	Femur	Malunion	External	Varus	Nail	YES	15.6	14.1	1.4	14.2	nonunion
5	F	32	Femur	Nonunion	Internal		Nail	YES	27.8	29.5	4.3	23.5	18
6	M	50	Femur	Malunion	External	Varus	Plate	none	20.2	20.3	-2.1	22.3	16
7	M	57	Femur	Nonunion	External		Nail	none	20	19.2	-4.2	24.2	18
8	M	70	Femur	Nonunion	Internal		Nail	YES	35.9	35.3	-3.3	39.2	20
9	M	57	Femur	Nonunion	External		Nail	YES	23.5	22.2	2.5	21	24
10	M	58	Femur	Nonunion	External		Nail	YES	11.2	10.4	-2.7	13.9	20
11	M	46	Femur	Nonunion	External		Nail	YES	23.9	23.4	4.8	19.1	18
12	M	11	Femur	Malalignment	Internal		Nail	none	20.6	20.1	-1.6	22.2	14
13	M	27	Femur	Nonunion	Internal		Nail	none	21.8	20.5	4.2	17.6	18
14	M	24	Femur	Malunion	Internal	Varus	Nail	none	17.8	19.6	3.0	14.8	16
15	F	15	Tibia	Malalignment	Internal	Procurvatum	Plate	none	16.3	14.7	1.3	15	14
16	M	77	Femur	Nonunion	External		Nail	none	23.1	20.2	4.6	18.5	20
17	M	17	Femur	Nonunion	External		Nail	YES	17.2	15.9	2.5	14.7	20
18	M	20	Tibia	Malunion	External		Nail	none	30.3	32.5	1.5	28.8	20
19	M	36	Femur	Nonunion	Internal		Nail	none	22.1	19.3	-1.8	23.9	18
		37.9							22.3	21.6	2.3	21.3	17.7

4. Discussion

Rotational osteotomy is a commonly used surgical treatment measure for the correction of malalignment caused by congenital, developmental, or posttraumatic factors. Techniques involving intraoperative fluoroscopic imaging have been used to ensure accurate correction, particularly along the coronal and sagittal planes. However, no reliable methods of assessing the intraoperative rotational alignment of the lower limbs have been reported to date. SP technology has been used previously in various orthopedic surgeries [18,19], with experimental studies examining its accuracy in the measurement of rotational deformities [14,15]. The findings were largely similar to those obtained using CT scanning with markers placed over artificial bones without any soft tissue coverage. However, angle measurement may be simpler in saw bone models as the markers are clearly visible, and this is in contrast to actual bony tissues in the extremities, which are typically enveloped by muscle and soft tissues that can interfere with visualization of the markers and prevent accurate measurement of angles. The findings of this study showed a strong correlation between angle-SP and postoperative angle-CT and, to the best of our knowledge, this is the first clinical series to examine derotational osteotomy and report accurate intraoperative measurement of correction using an SP app with an integrated gyroscope. Therefore, SP-assisted derotational osteotomy may be considered a suitable alternative for traditional osteotomies using open measuring.

Several fixation techniques for acute fractures also use fluoroscopic imaging to accurately measure rotation intraoperatively. They typically use anatomical landmarks (such as the lesser trochanter profile, patellar and fibular position, and native femoral torsion of the hip compared to the posterior femoral condylar plane) on the contralateral unaffected extremity as a template [20–22]. While these methods are also applicable in corrective osteotomy, variations in local anatomy may raise uncertainty regarding the accuracy of techniques based on visual estimation [23]. High rates of malrotation have been reported in patients with highly comminuted fractures, pre-existing anatomical deformities, or bilateral injuries [3,5]. Another limitation of techniques using fluoroscopy is the additional operative time required. Intraoperative use of mobile CT scanning [24,25] or computer navigation [26] is considered an ideal method for assessment of rotation, although their use is limited because of high associated costs, increased radiation exposure, and logistical issues in the operating room. In comparison, the proposed technique using an SP app measures the angle of rotation intuitively in real-time, is more economically viable, minimizes radiation exposure, and is also logistically convenient.

A recently introduced innovative surgical technique that corrects femoral malrotation using 3D printing technology [27] has the advantage of using customized cutting guides that allow accurate estimation of the angle of correction of malrotation. Additionally, it also requires shorter operating time and less radiation exposure. However, this technique requires a considerably invasive surgical approach as the 3D printed guides must be fixed proximal and distal to the osteotomy site, thus increasing the risk of blood loss, infection, and disturbed bone healing. Therefore, this technique may be unsuitable for the correction of postsurgical malalignment where the exposure of the previous fracture is unnecessary. In comparison, the proposed technique using SP app-assisted measurement requires minimal surgical exposure for percutaneous osteotomy and can even be carried out without opening the fracture site. Therefore, it allows for a less invasive approach, consequently reducing surgical morbidity and risk of infection. Additionally, it can also promote bone healing, as it allows preservation of the periosteal blood supply and the surrounding soft tissue. In the current study, 18 out of 19 patients exhibited primary bone healing without any infectious complications. Therefore, we believe that the proposed technique for derotational osteotomy sufficiently meets the requirement of minimal invasiveness.

Precise intraoperative measurement of the angle of derotation is important as it contributes to the functional outcomes after corrective osteotomy. Care should be taken to place markers during the procedure in order to allow accurate measurement of this parameter. After osteotomy, intraoperative measurement of the angle between the two markers is essential. A previous study examining version abnormalities of the femur used flat triangular osteotomy templates to estimate the angle between the markers visually [9]. However, its measurement may be rough and inaccurate, since the angles of triangles cannot match the different amount of the rotational malalignment. Although a sterilized goniometer may also be considered a suitable alternative, direct measurement may not be easy based on the distance between the markers. In comparison, the SP app can act as a customized alternative of the virtual goniometer that can determine the magnitude of rotational deformity precisely. This clinical trial showed a maximum difference of <5° between the affected and unaffected sides, suggesting that the use of a contemporary SP app is likely to achieve accuracy of measurement during derotational osteotomy.

Various operative techniques for correcting rotational deformities have been described in the literature. The conventional method is open exposure at the deformity level [28,29]. The correction angle is planned on preoperative CT scans and intraoperatively marked on the bone with Kirschner wires or Schanz screws. Subsequently, a transverse osteotomy and derotation are performed [28]. In our study, minimally invasive derotational osteotomy was carried out. This technique allows closed osteotomy without stripping the surrounding soft tissues, reducing surgical morbidity and risk of infection. The periosteum is left intact, which improves callus formation and bone healing. However, it is difficult to perform accurate angle correction, and there are disadvantages in that radiation exposure and intraoperative time increase. The proposed SP app technique can intuitively measure the rotation angle in real time and precisely determine the rotational deformity's magnitude. So, it can minimize radiation exposure and also decrease intraoperative time. However, the minimally invasive technique may be technically challenging surgery and requires a steep learning curve.

This study had several limitations, including a small sample size and no comparator groups. Future studies with a larger number of patients and appropriate comparison groups treated using other methods are necessary to confirm the efficacy of using the SP app for this purpose. This is the first study to carry out a large series of derotational osteotomies for the treatment of posttraumatic malalignments only. However, there are several factors that may affect the accuracy of measurement when using this technique. Firstly, errors may occur if the height and direction of the SP are not parallel to the two markers, emphasizing the need to ensure that the camera is placed on an imaginary line that is parallel to the markers when measuring. Secondly, errors may also occur if the markers are bent, with three patients in the current study exhibiting Schanz pins that were bent or broken during manual derotation. In such cases, reinsertion of the markers is essential if the fault is detected prior to measurement, and rotation of the distal limb should be carried out without holding the markers. Thirdly, loss of derotation during distal fixation of the implant can lead to over or undercorrection. An innovative technique using electromagnetic tracking (EMT) to monitor the angle of derotation continuously during surgery has been proposed previously [30]. However, this method is technically difficult and requires sterilization of specific parts (sensors or pointers) prior to use in the surgical setting. In comparison, the SP app does not require any complex equipment, and also offers minimal discrepancies between intraoperative derotation and postoperative results.

5. Conclusions

In conclusion, the SP app allows precise assessment of intraoperative angles during derotation osteotomy. SP app may help the newly introduced minimally invasive derotational osteotomy. It is a reliable and reproducible procedure to predict accurate angle measurement and produce excellent bone healing and function.

Author Contributions: Conceptualization: K.-H.P. and C.-W.O.; methodology: J.-W.K. (Joon-Woo Kim) and D.-H.K.; validation: S.-H.Y.; formal analysis: K.-H.P. and J.-H.L.; investigation: I.S. and C.-W.O.; data curation: I.S. and D.-H.K.; original draft preparation: K.-H.P. and C.-W.O.; draft review and editing: C.-W.O. and J.-W.K. (Joon-Woo Kim); visualization: K.-H.P. and S.-H.Y.; supervision: C.-W.O. and J.-W.K. (Ji-Wan Kim). All authors have read and agreed to the published version of the manuscript.

Funding: This work was supported by a Biomedical Research Institute grant, Kyungpook National University Hospital (2020).

Institutional Review Board Statement: The design and protocol of this study were approved by the institutional review board of Kyungpook National University Hospital (IRB no: KNUH 2020-11-009, approved on 4 December 2020).

Informed Consent Statement: Informed consent was obtained from all individual participants included in this study.

Data Availability Statement: Source data may be shared by the corresponding author upon reasonable request.

Conflicts of Interest: The authors declare no conflict of interest.

References

1. Greco, T.; Cianni, L.; Polichetti, C.; Inverso, M.; Maccauro, G.; Perisano, C. Uncoated vs. Antibiotic-Coated Tibia Nail in Open Diaphyseal Tibial Fracture (42 according to AO Classification): A Single Center Experience. *BioMed Res. Int.* **2021**, *2021*, 7421582. [CrossRef]
2. Perisano, C.; Cianni, L.; Polichetti, C.; Cannella, A.; Mosca, M.; Caravelli, S.; Maccauro, G.; Greco, T. Plate Augmentation in Aseptic Femoral Shaft Nonunion after Intramedullary Nailing: A Literature Review. *Bioengineering* **2022**, *9*, 560. [CrossRef]
3. Jaarsma, R.L.; Pakvis, D.F.M.; Verdonschot, N.; Biert, J.; Van Kampen, A. Rotational Malalignment After Intramedullary Nailing of Femoral Fractures. *J. Orthop. Trauma* **2004**, *18*, 403–409. [CrossRef]
4. Karaman, O.; Ayhan, E.; Kesmezacar, H.; Seker, A.; Unlu, M.C.; Aydingoz, O. Rotational malalignment after closed intramedullary nailing of femoral shaft fractures and its influence on daily life. *Eur. J. Orthop. Surg. Traumatol.* **2014**, *24*, 1243–1247. [CrossRef]
5. Kim, J.-W.; Oh, C.-W.; Oh, J.-K.; Park, I.-H.; Kyung, H.-S.; Park, K.-H.; Yoon, S.-D.; Kim, S.-M. Malalignment after minimally invasive plate osteosynthesis in distal femoral fractures. *Injury* **2017**, *48*, 751–757. [CrossRef]
6. Çepni, Ş.; Yaman, F.; Veizi, E.; Fırat, A.; Çay, N.; Tecimel, O. Does Malrotation After Minimally Invasive Plate Osteosynthesis Treatment of Distal Tibia Metaphyseal Fractures Effect the Functional Results of the Ankle and Knee Joints? *J. Orthop. Trauma* **2021**, *35*, 492–498. [CrossRef]
7. Boscher, J.; Alain, A.; Vergnenegre, G.; Hummel, V.; Charissoux, J.-L.; Marcheix, P.-S. Femoral shaft fractures treated by antegrade locked intramedullary nailing: EOS stereoradiographic imaging evaluation of rotational malalignment having a functional impact. *Orthop. Traumatol. Surg. Res.* **2022**, *108*, 103235. [CrossRef] [PubMed]
8. Nelitz, M. Femoral derotational osteotomies. *Curr. Rev. Musculoskelet. Med.* **2018**, *11*, 272–279. [CrossRef] [PubMed]
9. Buly, R.L.; Sosa, B.R.; Poultsides, L.A.; Caldwell, E.; Rozbruch, S.R. Femoral Derotation Osteotomy in Adults for Version Abnormalities. *J. Am. Acad. Orthop. Surg.* **2018**, *26*, e416–e425. [CrossRef] [PubMed]
10. Lee, H.-J.; Oh, C.-W.; Kim, J.-W.; Jung, J.-W.; Park, B.-C.; Song, K.-S. Rotational osteotomy with submuscular plating in skeletally immature patients with cerebral palsy. *J. Orthop. Sci.* **2013**, *18*, 557–562. [CrossRef]
11. Zeckey, C.; Bogusch, M.; Borkovec, M.; Becker, C.A.; Neuerburg, C.; Weidert, S.; Suero, E.M.; Böcker, W.; Greiner, A.; Kammerlander, C. Radiographic cortical thickness parameters as predictors of rotational alignment in proximal femur fractures: A cadaveric study. *J. Orthop. Res.* **2019**, *37*, 69–76. [CrossRef] [PubMed]
12. Degen, N.; Suero, E.; Bogusch, M.; Neuerburg, C.; Manz, K.M.; Becker, C.A.; Befrui, N.; Kammerlander, C.; Böcker, W.; Zeckey, C. Intraoperative use of cortical step sign and diameter difference sign: Accuracy, inter-rater agreement and influence of surgical experience in subtrochanteric transverse fractures. *Orthop. Traumatol. Surg. Res.* **2020**, *106*, 639–644. [CrossRef] [PubMed]
13. Fang, C.; Gibson, W.; Lau, T.W.; Fang, B.; Wong, T.M.; Leung, F. Important tips and numbers on using the cortical step and diameter difference sign in assessing femoral rotation—Should we abandon the technique? *Injury* **2015**, *46*, 1393–1399. [CrossRef] [PubMed]
14. Graham, D.; Suzuki, A.; Reitz, C.; Saxena, A.; Kuo, J.; Tetsworth, K. Measurement of rotational deformity: Using a smartphone application is more accurate than conventional methods. *ANZ J. Surg.* **2013**, *83*, 937–941. [CrossRef]
15. Shen, Y.; Huang, J.; Li, X.; Gao, H. Evaluation of the smartphone for measurement of femoral rotational deformity. *ANZ J. Surg.* **2019**, *89*, E422–E427. [CrossRef]
16. Yoon, R.S.; Koerner, J.D.; Patel, N.M.; Sirkin, M.S.; Reilly, M.C.; Liporace, F.A. Impact of specialty and level of training on CT measurement of femoral version: An interobserver agreement analysis. *J. Orthop. Traumatol.* **2013**, *14*, 277–281. [CrossRef]

17. Bleeker, N.J.; Cain, M.; Rego, M.; Saarig, A.; Chan, A.; Sierevelt, I.; Doornberg, J.N.; Jaarsma, R.L. Bilateral Low-Dose Computed Tomography Assessment for Post-Operative Rotational Malalignment After Intramedullary Nailing for Tibial Shaft Fractures: Reliability of a Practical Imaging Technique. *Injury* **2018**, *49*, 1895–1900. [CrossRef]
18. Kamimura, A.; Enokida, M.; Enokida, S.; Nagashima, H. A method combining the use of a mobile application and a dedicated pelvic positioner for acetabular cup insertion. *J. Orthop. Surg. Res.* **2022**, *17*, 251. [CrossRef]
19. Peters, F.M.; Greeff, R.; Goldstein, N.; Frey, C.T. Improving Acetabular Cup Orientation in Total Hip Arthroplasty by Using Smartphone Technology. *J. Arthroplast.* **2012**, *27*, 1324–1330. [CrossRef]
20. Cain, M.E.; Hendrickx, L.A.M.; Bleeker, N.J.; Lambers, K.T.A.; Doornberg, J.N.; Jaarsma, R.L. Prevalence of rotational malalignment after intramedullary nailing of tibial shaft fractures: Can we reliably use the contralateral uninjured side as the reference standard? *J. Bone Jt. Surg. Am.* **2020**, *102*, 582–591. [CrossRef]
21. Krettek, C.; Miclau, T.; Grün, O.; Schandelmaier, P.; Tscherne, H. Intraoperative control of axes, rotation and length in femoral and tibial fractures technical note. *Injury* **1998**, *29* (Suppl. S3), 29–39. [CrossRef]
22. Tornetta, P.; Ritz, G.; Kantor, A. Femoral Torsion after Interlocked Nailing of Unstable Femoral Fractures. *J. Trauma Inj. Infect. Crit. Care* **1995**, *38*, 213–219. [CrossRef] [PubMed]
23. Marchand, L.S.; Todd, D.C.; Kellam, P.; Adeyemi, T.F.; Rothberg, D.L.; Maak, T.G. Is the lesser trochanter profile a reliable means of restoring anatomic rotation after femur fracture fixation? *Clin. Orthop. Relat. Res.* **2018**, *476*, 1253–1261. [CrossRef] [PubMed]
24. Hawi, N.; Liodakis, E.; Suero, E.M.; Stuebig, T.; Citak, M.; Krettek, C. Radiological outcome and intraoperative evaluation of a computer-navigation system for femoral nailing: A retrospective cohort study. *Injury* **2014**, *45*, 1632–1636. [CrossRef] [PubMed]
25. Ramme, A.J.; Egol, J.; Chang, G.; Davidovitch, R.I.; Konda, S. Evaluation of malrotation following intramedullary nailing in a femoral shaft fracture model: Can a 3d c-arm improve accuracy? *Injury* **2017**, *48*, 1603–1608. [CrossRef] [PubMed]
26. Wilharm, A.; Gras, F.; Rausch, S.; Linder, R.; Marintschev, I.; Hofmann, G.; Mückley, T. Navigation in femoral-shaft fractures—From lab tests to clinical routine. *Injury* **2011**, *42*, 1346–1352. [CrossRef]
27. Oraa, J.; Beitia, M.; Fiz, N.; González, S.; Sánchez, X.; Delgado, D.; Sánchez, M. Custom 3D-Printed Cutting Guides for Femoral Osteotomy in Rotational Malalignment Due to Diaphyseal Fractures: Surgical Technique and Case Series. *J. Clin. Med.* **2021**, *10*, 3366. [CrossRef]
28. Kreusch-Brinker, R.; Schwetlick, G. Korrekturosteotomien an Femur- und Tibiaschaft mit dem Verriegelungsnagel [Corrective osteotomy of the femoral and tibial shafts using the interlocking nail]. *Unfallchirurgie* **1990**, *16*, 236–243. [CrossRef]
29. Zenker, H. Zur Indikation und Technik korrigierender Osteotomien im Schaftbereich langer Röhrenknochen [Indications and technic of correction osteotomies in the shaft of long bones]. *Arch. Orthop. Unfallchir.* **1972**, *74*, 205–223. [CrossRef]
30. Geisbüsch, A.; Auer, C.; Dickhaus, H.; Niklasch, M.; Dreher, T. Electromagnetic bone segment tracking to control femoral derotation osteotomy—A saw bone study. *J. Orthop. Res.* **2017**, *35*, 1106–1112. [CrossRef]

Disclaimer/Publisher's Note: The statements, opinions and data contained in all publications are solely those of the individual author(s) and contributor(s) and not of MDPI and/or the editor(s). MDPI and/or the editor(s) disclaim responsibility for any injury to people or property resulting from any ideas, methods, instructions or products referred to in the content.

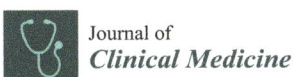

Article

Relationships between Jumping Performance and Psychological Readiness to Return to Sport 6 Months Following Anterior Cruciate Ligament Reconstruction: A Cross-Sectional Study

Claudio Legnani [1,*], Matteo Del Re [2], Marco Viganò [3], Giuseppe M. Peretti [3,4], Enrico Borgo [1] and Alberto Ventura [1]

1. Sport Traumatology and Minimally Invasive Surgery Center, IRCCS Istituto Ortopedico Galeazzi, 20161 Milan, Italy
2. Department of Orthopedics and Traumatology, University of Milan, 20133 Milan, Italy
3. IRCCS Istituto Ortopedico Galeazzi, 20161 Milan, Italy
4. Department of Biomedical Sciences for Health, University of Milan, 20133 Milan, Italy
* Correspondence: claudio.legnani@grupposandonato.it

Abstract: Background: Investigating the relationship between functional capacity and psychological readiness is of paramount importance when planning sport resumption following knee surgery. The aim of this study was to prospectively assess clinical and functional outcomes in athletes 6 months after primary anterior cruciate ligament (ACL) reconstruction and to evaluate whether jumping ability is related to psychological readiness to return to sport following ACL surgery. Methods: Patients who underwent ACL reconstruction were prospectively enrolled and evaluated pre-operatively and 6 months after surgery. Assessment included Lysholm score, International Knee Documentation Committee (IKDC) Subjective Knee Form, Tegner activity level, and the ACL–Return to Sport after Injury (ACL-RSI) scale. Jumping ability was instrumentally assessed by an infrared optical acquisition system using a test battery including mono- and bipodalic vertical jump and a side hop test. Patients were dichotomized by ACL-RSI into two groups: group A (ACL-RSI > 60), and group B (ACL-RSI < 60). Results: Overall, 29 males and two females from the original study group of 37 patients (84%) were available for clinical evaluation. Mean age at surgery was 34.2 years (SD 11.3). Mean body mass index (BMI) was 25.4 (SD 3.7). Mean overall Lysholm, IKDC, and ACL-RSI scores increased from pre-operatively ($p < 0.001$). No differences in Tegner score were reported ($p = 0.161$). Similarly, improvement in most variables regarding jumping ability were observed at follow-up ($p < 0.05$). According to ACL-RSI, 20 subjects were allocated in group A (ACL-RSI > 60), while 11 were allocated in group B (ACL-RSI < 60). A statistically significant difference in favor of patients in group A was recorded for the post-operative Lysholm and Tegner score, as well as Side Hop test LSI level ($p < 0.05$), while a trend for IKDC was observed without statistical significance ($p = 0.065$). Conclusions: Patients with higher values of ACL-RSI scores showed better functional and clinical outcomes as well as improved performance 6 months after ACL reconstruction

Keywords: anterior cruciate ligament; ACL reconstruction; return to sports; ACL-RSI; psychological readiness; vertical jump

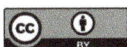

1. Introduction

The treatment of anterior cruciate ligament (ACL) rupture in the physically active population is often surgical. Patients treated with ACL reconstruction usually aim to return to sport activities they practiced before injury [1–3].

However, a significant number of patients ranging between 37% and 56% are not able to return to sport at pre-injury level [4]. Reasons for that include the persistence of knee strength and neuromuscular deficits, kinesiophobia, and fear of re-injury [5]. Increased risks of re-rupture have been reported within the first two years after surgery, especially in the youngest patients [6,7]. For these reasons, in an attempt to reduce risk factors and to determine the appropriate timing for resuming sports activities, test batteries have been developed. These include but are not limited to jumping abilities assessment, strength tests, and psychological readiness scoring systems [8–11]. Tests measuring muscular power and reactivity through vertical jump are demonstrated to be reliable instruments and useful predictors for the return to sports [11,12]. Horizontal hop tests have been widely adopted to detect functional asymmetries between limbs [13,14], although their usefulness has been questioned as they are demonstrated to overestimate the involved limb's function following ACL surgery [15,16]. Investigating the relationship between functional capacity and psychological readiness is of paramount importance when planning sport resumption following ACL reconstruction [9]. Therefore, vertical jump tests have been advocated to better analyze knee biomechanics, thus identifying lower limb asymmetries more accurately, and give a more reliable prediction on the return-to-sport ability [11].

The ACL–Return to Sport after Injury scale (ACL-RSI) is considered a reliable tool to assess psychological readiness to return to sport after ACL surgery [17,18]. It has been demonstrated that patients with lower ACL-RSI scores are at higher risk for ACL re-rupture [19], and recently much emphasis is given to the recovery of psychological responses as a criterion used to clear athletes to return to sport following ACL reconstruction.

The aim of this study was to prospectively assess outcomes of athletes who had undergone primary ACL reconstruction at 6 months after surgery, and to evaluate whether psychological readiness affects functional and clinical results as well as jumping ability. The hypothesis was that athletes' psychological readiness is strictly related to jumping performance.

2. Materials and Methods

2.1. Patient Recruitment

From January 2021 to the end of December 2021, 37 consecutive patients who underwent ACL reconstruction at the Department of Sport Traumatology and Minimally Invasive Surgery of our Institution were prospectively enrolled and evaluated pre-operatively and 6 months after surgery. Diagnosis was done with clinical examination and knee magnetic resonance imaging, and further verified arthroscopically. All surgeries were performed by the same senior surgeon.

Inclusion criteria were: primary unilateral ACL reconstruction; age $\geq$ 18 years and $\leq$45 years at surgery; time from injury to surgery $\geq$ 2 weeks and $\leq$12 months; participation in sporting activity; same postoperative rehabilitation protocol. Exclusion criteria were: past history of ligamental surgery on the same or contralateral knee; concomitant surgical procedures with the exception of treatment for meniscal pathology; pregnancy; inability to complete clinical and functional testing.

The study received Institutional Review Board approval (IRB number: 57/INT/2020, released from IRCCS San Raffaele Hospital, Milan, Italy). All participants signed informed consent.

2.2. Surgical Technique and Rehabilitation Protocol

All patients underwent arthroscopic-assisted ACL reconstruction using doubled autologous hamstring graft [6]. Tibial tunnel was drilled using a 55° guide (Acufex; Smith & Nephew, Andover, MA, USA) using as reference the posterior cruciate ligament, while the femoral half-tunnel was prepared either through the medial portal or with a trans-tibial technique. Fixation was achieved proximally with a cortical suspension device (Retrobutton; Arthrex Inc., Naples, FL, USA) and distally through a bioadsorbable interference screw (Milagro; DePuy Mitek, Raynham, MA, USA). A brace-free rehabilitation protocol starting the day after surgery was adopted in all patients, with immediate regaining of extension, isometric exercises, and walking with crutches with partial weight bearing for the first 3 weeks. Swimming and indoor cycling were allowed after 12 weeks, while after 5 months a protocol of jump technique training and plyometric exercises was started.

2.3. Follow-Up Assessment

Assessment included Lysholm score, International Knee Documentation Committee (IKDC) Subjective Knee Form, Tegner activity level, and ACL-RSI scale. The Lysholm score is a 100-point maximum subjective questionnaire developed to evaluate knee functional status after ACL surgery [20]. The IKDC subjective score is a clinical questionnaire that assesses the functional status of the knee ranging from 0 to 100, with 100 indicating no limitations [21]. The Tegner activity scale is designed to grade patient's activity level based on work and sports activities from 0 (lowest level) to 10 [22]. ACL-RSI is a previously validated 12-item questionnaire that allows evaluating psychological readiness to return to sport following ACL injury or surgery on a scale from 0 to 100. The Italian version of the ACL-RSI used in the present study showed excellent internal consistency and reliability [18].

Jumping ability was assessed using a test battery modified from Gustavsson et al. [23], using the OptoGait (Microgate, Bolzano, Italy) system. This device allows us to calculate jumping height (in centimeters) from flight time (in milliseconds) measured by an infrared optical acquisition system connected to a software (OptoGait analysis software, version 3.22; Microgate).

Two types of bipodalic jumps were tested: squat jump (SJ), and countermovement jump (CMJ) (Figures 1 and 2). Then, monopodalic jumps were performed: CMJ, and side hop test (Figures 3 and 4). Each of them was performed with the uninjured limb first, followed by the injured. The SJ consisted of a vertical jump performed from a half-squat position with the knees flexed at 90°. The CMJ was performed in the same fashion, with the exception that the starting position was an upright position, and the jump was performed after a quick sinking. Every jump was performed 3 times, and the average value was recorded. The side hop test consisted of performing as many jumps as possible during a period of 30 s between two parallel strips on the floor put at a distance of 30 cm without touching the strips (a maximum of 25% error was allowed; otherwise, the test was repeated). Limb Symmetry Index (LSI) was calculated as a percentage of test performance on the injured/operated limb compared to the contralateral limb.

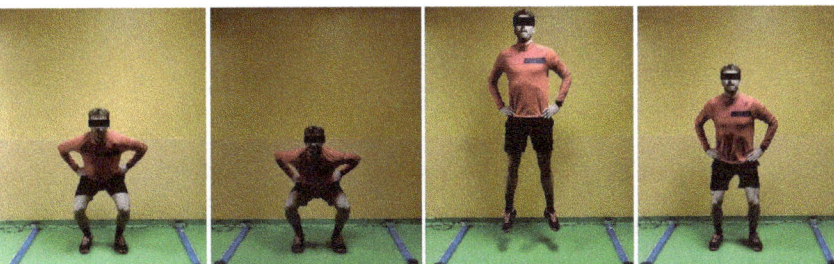

Figure 1. Bipodalic squat jump.

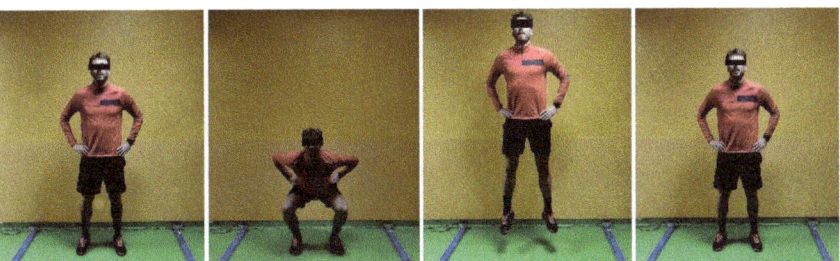

Figure 2. Bipodalic countermovement jump.

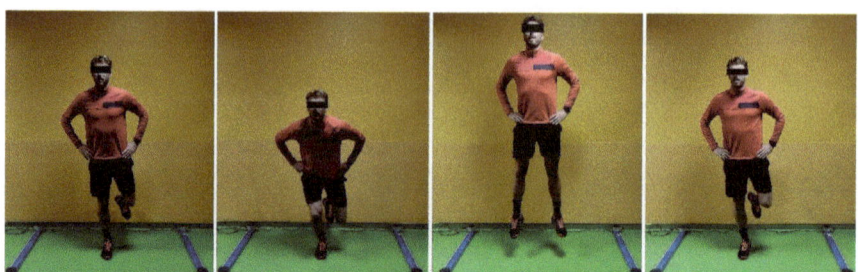

Figure 3. Monopodalic countermovement jump.

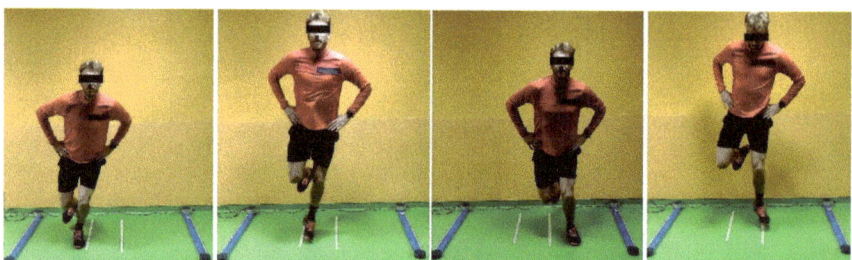

Figure 4. Monopodalic side hop test.

2.4. Statistical Analysis

Statistical analyses were performed using Graphpad Prism v8.0 (Prism software, La Jolla, San Diego, CA, USA). Shapiro–Wilk test was used to test the distribution of each variable. In case of normal distribution, paired Student t tests were used to assess differences between pre-operative and 6-month values. Patients were dichotomized by post-operative ACL-RSI score into two groups: group A (ACL-RSI > 60), and group B (ACL-RSI < 60); unpaired t test were used to evaluate differences between the two groups. In case of non-normal distribution, the same assessments were performed by Wilcoxon signed-rank test for matched pairs and Mann–Whitney U test, respectively. Difference between proportions were assessed by Fisher's exact test. p values < 0.05 were considered statistically significant. Post-hoc power analysis was performed for the test evaluating the improvements in Lysholm, ACL-RSI, and IKDC after surgery. For a test with alpha = 0.05, the study sample size provided a test power > 90% for each score.

3. Results

3.1. Demographic Data

Six patients (16%) were lost at follow-up. Overall, there were 29 males and two females available for clinical evaluation. Mean age at surgery was 34.2 years (SD 11.3). Mean body mass index (BMI) was 25.4 (SD 3.7). Average time interval between injury to surgery was 2.7 months (SD: 1.1). Patients' demographics and anthropometric data are reported in Table 1. At the time of injury, 21 patients practiced contact sports (soccer, basketball, rugby). Noncontact sports (volleyball, skiing, cycling, running, swimming, tennis) were practiced in 28 cases. Eleven patients practiced sport at an agonistic level, 20 were amateurs.

Table 1. Patient demographics and anthropometric data.

	Overall	ACL-RSI > 60	ACL-RSI < 60	p-Value
No. of patients	31	20	11	
Gender				
Male	29	19	10	
Female	2	1	1	
Mean ACL-RSI score (SD)	68.3 (16.2)	78.2 (9.1)	50.2 (8.5)	
Mean age at surgery (SD) (yr)	34.6 (11.7)	34.7 (11.4)	34.4 (12.5)	0.9
Mean BMI (SD)	25.1 (3.2)	25.4 (3.4)	24.5 (2.7)	0.4

ACL-RSI: Anterior Cruciate Ligament Return to Sport after Injury; SD: standard deviation; BMI: Body Mass.

3.2. Subjective Knee Function

The mean overall Lysholm score increased from a pre-operative mean of 68.4 (SD: 15.6) to 87.1 (SD: 11.2), showing a statistically significant difference ($p < 0.001$). IKDC subjective score improved from 51.9 (SD: 13.0) to 77.1 (SD: 14.6) ($p < 0.001$). Similarly, ACL-RSI changed from 46.2 (SD: 23.2) to 68.3 (SD: 16.2) ($p < 0.001$). Concerning Tegner activity level, no statistically significant differences were reported between pre- and post-operative status (mean value 4.2, SD: 2.4, and 5.1, SD: 1.8, respectively, $p = 0.161$) (Table 2, Figure 5).

Table 2. Overall comparison between pre-operative and follow-up status.

	Pre-Operative	Follow-Up	p-Value
Lysholm score (mean, SD)	68.4 (15.6)	87.1 (11.2)	<0.001
Mean ACL-RSI score (SD)	51.9 (13.0)	77.1 (14.6)	<0.001
Mean age at surgery (SD) (yr)	46.2 (23.2)	68.3 (16.2)	<0.001
Tegner activity level (mean, SD)	4.2 (2.4)	5.1 (1.8)	0.161

SD: standard deviation; IKDC: International Knee Documentation Committee; ACL-RSI: Anterior Cruciate Ligament Return to Sport after Injury.

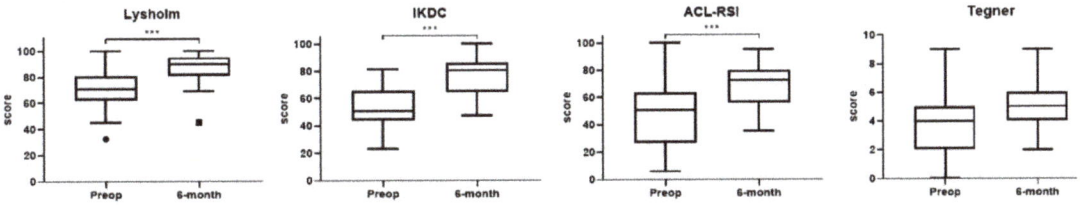

Figure 5. Box-plots showing differences in outcome scores from pre-operative to 6-month follow-up after surgery. The black line inside the box represents median value. The lowest bar represents the minimum value, the bottom and top of the boxes represent the interquartile range (25th and 75th percentiles), and the top bar represents the maximum value. Points outside the limits represent outliers *** $p < 0.001$.

3.3. Jump Battery Tests

The following variables significantly improved at follow-up compared to pre-operatory status: bipodalic CMJ ($p = 0.049$), monopodalic CMJ on the injured limb ($p = 0.037$), CMJ LSI ($p = 0.037$), 30 s Side Hop test on the injured limb ($p < 0.001$), and Side Hop test LSI ($p < 0.001$) (Figure 6). No differences in other jump tests were recorded ($p = $ n.s.).

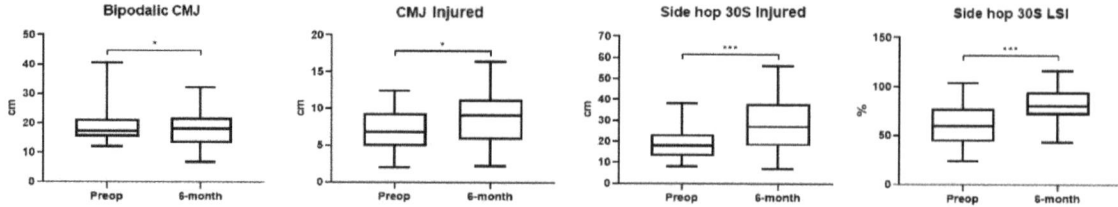

Figure 6. Box-plots showing differences in jumping performances from pre-operative to 6-month follow-up after surgery. The black line inside the box represents median value. The lowest bar represents the minimum value, the bottom and top of the boxes represent the interquartile range (25th and 75th percentiles), and the top bar represents the maximum value. * $p < 0.05$; *** $p < 0.001$.

3.4. Results According to ACL-RSI

Patients were dichotomized by post-operative ACL-RSI into two groups: 20 subjects were allocated in group A (ACL-RSI > 60), while 11 were allocated in group B (ACL-RSI < 60). No statistically significant differences between these two groups were reported concerning average Lysholm, IKDC, ACL-RSI, and Tegner score ($p = 0.92$, 0.69, 0.21, and 0.44, respectively) at baseline.

Between groups, comparisons were performed using individual changes with respect to baseline, in order to adjust for possible biases. A statistically significant difference in favour of group A was recorded for Lysholm score ($p = 0.020$) and Tegner activity level ($p = 0.006$), while a trend for IKDC was observed without statistical significance ($p = 0.065$) (Figure 7). Considering jump tests, the following variable was significantly higher in group A: Side Hop test LSI ($p < 0.05$) (Figure 8). No differences concerning other jump tests were recorded between the two groups (p = n.s.).

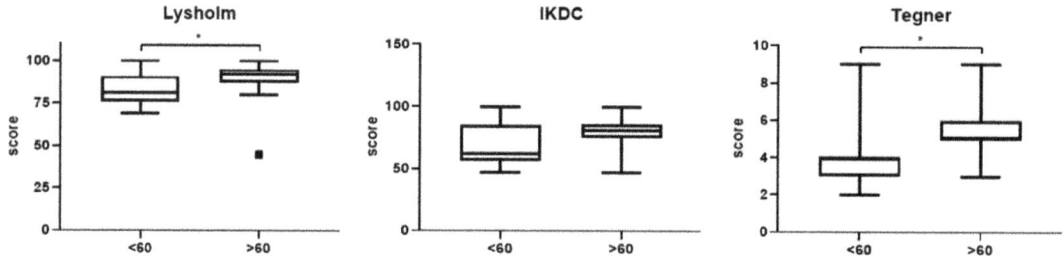

Figure 7. Box-plots showing differences between the two groups with the same change compared to the baseline for the various parameters. The black line inside the box represents median value. The lowest bar represents the 10th percentile, the bottom and top of the boxes represent the interquartile range (25th and 75th percentiles), and the top bar represents the 90th percentile. * $p < 0.05$.

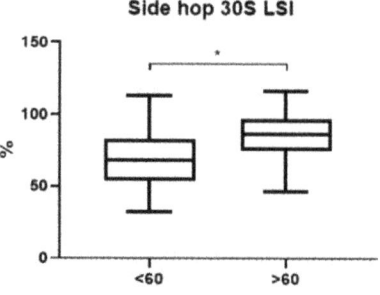

Figure 8. Box-plot showing differences in Side Hop test LSI between the two groups. The black

line inside the box represents median value. The lowest bar represents the minimum value, the bottom and top of the box represent the interquartile range (25th and 75th percentiles), and the top bar represents the maximum value. * $p < 0.05$.

4. Discussion

The most important finding of the present study was that patients with higher values of ACL-RSI scores showed better functional clinical outcomes according to Lysholm and Tegner scores as well as improved performance as measured with side-hop test six months after ACL reconstruction.

According to our results, six months after surgery, subjective knee function according to point-scales significantly improved compared to pre-operatory status, thus supporting the efficacy of hamstring ACL reconstruction in athletes.

Functional tests are commonly used to assess the return-to-sport ability following ACL reconstruction. In our cohort of patients, a test battery of vertical jumps measured with an optical acquisition equipment was adopted to evaluate jump performance following ACL surgery. Assessment of vertical jump to detect function deficits of the lower limb with ACL injury or following ACL surgery has been previously reported [11,12,24]. The battery of vertical jump tests used in the present investigation involved bipodalic SJ, bipodalic and monopodalic CMJs, and 30 s side hop test. Such tests, by measuring jump height as an expression of knee explosiveness, coordination, and dynamic knee stability, are reliable predictors for the return to sport after ACL surgery. Based on the results of these test batteries, LSI was calculated to evaluate knee status and patient ability to return to cutting and pivoting sports.

Six months after surgery, the ability to perform bipodalic CMJ, monopodalic CMJ on the injured limb, and a 30 s Side Hop test on the injured limb significantly improved at follow-up compared to pre-operatory status. Similarly, an improvement in LSI recorded while performing CMJ and Side Hop test LSI was observed.

Previous studies investigated the relationship between psychological readiness and functional performance [13,25,26]. The ACL-RSI score demonstrated to be a reliable scoring scale while evaluating psychological readiness for return to sports after ACL reconstruction [17,18]. In the study by McPherson et al., patients who underwent ACL re-rupture trended toward lower ACL-RSI scores [19], while according to Sadeqi et al., ACL-RSI score $\geq$ 60 months after surgery is a reliable predictor of return to preinjury sport [27]. According to the study by Aizawa et al., in our case series, we considered 60 as a cut-off value to evaluate psychologic readiness to return to sport six months after surgery [13]. Webster et al. followed up with 635 athletes 12 months after ACL reconstruction, and observed that greater limb symmetry while performing a single-legged hop for distance positively correlates with the ACL-RSI score [26]. Similarly, in the study by Aizawa et al. on athletes aiming to return to sport participation six months after surgery, LSI while performing jump tests affected the ACL-RSI score [25].

According to our findings, using individual changes with respect to baseline, patients with ACL-RSI score > 60 reported higher Lysholm and Tegner score and higher performance in the side-hop test six months after ACL surgery compared to patients with ACL-RSI score < 60. Sport-related performances such as vertical jump following ACL reconstruction are affected by muscular co-ordination recovery, leg power, and symmetry in isokinetic lower limb strength. Our study demonstrated that the ability to perform a side-hop test was significantly higher in the group with better psychological readiness. Similarly, patients with higher confidence tended towards higher PROMs compared to patients not meeting the ACL-RSI threshold of 60 points. This confirms our hypothesis that psychological readiness is strictly related to jumping ability. Interestingly, no difference with respect to subjective IKDC score, SJ, and CMJs were reported between the two groups considered.

Further research is needed to investigate the most reliable predictors affecting ACL-RSI score at the time of return to sport.

Return to pre-injury activity level represents one of the most important issues in patients following ACL reconstruction. According to our results, average activity level did not statistically differ from pre-operative at follow-up, thus supporting the findings that most patients return to pre-injury activity level up to 12 months after surgery [28].

Future studies should build on current preliminary findings to help to evaluate return-to-sport readiness following ACL surgery, taking into account functional ability and psychological readiness when planning sport resumption. Long-term studies are needed to investigate prognostic factors which may allow for more appropriate decision-making strategies and give a reliable prediction on return-to-sport ability [29,30].

This study possesses limitations. The relatively small sample size may not have allowed for the detection of small differences between groups regarding some parameters. A trend for increased IKDC score in patients with ACL-RSI > 60 failed to demonstrate statistical significance. A greater number of patients could have enhanced the power of the results obtained. We acknowledge that jumping ability is influenced by many variables, and correlating jump height with neuromuscular restoration following ACL surgery is a further study limitation. The OptoGait device was chosen to instrumentally assess jump performance because it is simple, relatively inexpensive, and easily reproducible in the clinical setting allowing us to perform reliable measurements of functional ability. The male/female ratio of the patients recruited was biased towards the male gender, therefore our findings may not be generalizable to female athletes. Another limitation was the lack of a control group of healthy individuals. Finally, relying on subjective questionnaires could potentially bias the results. Long-term prospective follow-up studies with larger cohorts are required to corroborate these findings.

5. Conclusions

Patients with higher values of ACL-RSI scores showed better functional and clinical outcomes as well as improved performance six months after ACL reconstruction. Psychological readiness to return to sport reflects a better recovery of knee function following ACL surgery.

Author Contributions: Conceptualization, A.V.; methodology, C.L. and M.D.R.; software, M.V.; validation, C.L. and E.B.; formal analysis, C.L., M.V. and M.D.R.; investigation, M.D.R.; resources, A.V. and E.B.; data curation, C.L., M.V. and M.D.R.; writing—original draft preparation, C.L.; writing—review and editing, A.V. and G.M.P.; visualization, C.L.; supervision, A.V. and G.M.P.; project administration, A.V.; funding acquisition, C.L. and A.V. All authors have read and agreed to the published version of the manuscript.

Funding: This research was funded by the Italian Ministry of Health.

Institutional Review Board Statement: The study was conducted in accordance with the Declaration of Helsinki. The study received Institutional Review Board approval (IRB number: 57/INT/2020, released from IRCCS San Raffaele Hospital, Milan, Italy).

Informed Consent Statement: Informed consent was obtained from all participants involved in the study.

Data Availability Statement: Raw data will be provided on request.

Conflicts of Interest: The authors declare no conflict of interest.

References

1. McCullough, K.A.; Phelps, K.D.; Spindler, K.P.; Matava, M.J.; Dunn, W.R.; Parker, R.D.; Group, M.; Reinke, E.K. Return to high school- and college-level football after anterior cruciate ligament reconstruction: A Multicenter Orthopaedic Outcomes Network (MOON) cohort study. *Am. J. Sports Med.* **2012**, *49*, 2523–2529. [CrossRef] [PubMed]
2. Ardern, C.L.; Taylor, N.F.; Feller, J.A.; Webster, K.E. Return-to-sport outcomes at 2 to 7 years after anterior cruciate ligament reconstruction surgery. *Am. J. Sports Med.* **2012**, *40*, 41–48. [CrossRef] [PubMed]

3. Pinheiro, V.H.; Jones, M.; Borque, K.A.; Balendra, G.; White, N.P.; Ball, S.V.; Williams, A. Rates and Levels of Elite Sport Participation at 5 Years after Revision ACL Reconstruction. *Am. J. Sports Med.* **2022**, *50*, 3762–3769. [CrossRef]
4. Ardern, C.L.; Webster, K.E.; Taylor, N.F.; Feller, J.A. Return to sport following anterior cruciate ligament reconstruction surgery: A systematic review and meta-analysis on the state of play. *Br. J. Sports Med.* **2011**, *45*, 596–606. [CrossRef] [PubMed]
5. Webster, K.E.; Feller, J.A. A research update on the state of play for return to sport after anterior cruciate ligament reconstruction. *J. Orthop. Traumatol.* **2019**, *20*, 10. [CrossRef] [PubMed]
6. Legnani, C.; Peretti, G.M.; Del Re, M.; Borgo, E.; Ventura, A. Return to sports and re-rupture rate following anterior cruciate ligament reconstruction in amateur sportsman: Long-term outcomes. *J. Sports Med. Phys. Fitness* **2019**, *59*, 1902–1907. [CrossRef]
7. Zhao, D.; Pan, J.K.; Lin, F.Z.; Luo, M.H.; Liang, G.H.; Zeng, L.F.; Huang, H.T.; Han, Y.H.; Xu, N.J.; Yang, W.Y.; et al. Risk Factors for Revision or Rerupture After Anterior Cruciate Ligament Reconstruction: A Systematic Review and Meta-analysis. *Am. J. Sports Med.* **2022**, *3*, 3635465221119787. [CrossRef]
8. Crotty, N.M.N.; Daniels, K.A.J.; McFadden, C.; Cafferkey, N.; King, E. Relationship Between Isokinetic Knee Strength and Single-Leg Drop Jump Performance 9 Months after ACL Reconstruction. *Orthop. J. Sports Med.* **2022**, *10*, 23259671211063800. [CrossRef]
9. Turk, R.; Shah, S.; Chilton, M.; Thomas, T.L.; Anene, C.; Mousad, A.; Le Breton, S.; Li, L.; Pettit, R.; Ives, K.; et al. Critical Criteria Recommendations: Return to Sport After ACL reconstruction requires evaluation of time after surgery of 8 months, >2 functional tests, psychological readiness, and quadriceps/hamstring strength. *Arthroscopy* **2022**. [CrossRef]
10. Chona, D.; Eriksson, K.; Young, S.W.; Denti, M.; Sancheti, P.K.; Safran, M.; Sherman, S. Return to sport following anterior cruciate ligament reconstruction: The argument for a multimodal approach to optimise decision-making: Current concepts. *J. ISAKOS* **2021**, *6*, 344–348. [CrossRef]
11. Kotsifaki, A.; Van Rossom, S.; Whiteley, R.; Korakakis, V.; Bahr, R.; Sideris, V.; Jonkers, I. Single leg vertical jump performance identifies knee function deficits at return to sport after ACL reconstruction in male athletes. *Br. J. Sports Med.* **2022**, *56*, 490–498. [CrossRef] [PubMed]
12. Ventura, A.; Iori, S.; Legnani, C.; Terzaghi, C.; Borgo, E.; Albisetti, W. Single-bundle versus double-bundle anterior cruciate ligament reconstruction: Assessment with vertical jump test. *Arthroscopy* **2013**, *29*, 1201–1210. [CrossRef] [PubMed]
13. Aizawa, J.; Hirohata, K.; Ohji, S.; Ohmi, T.; Mitomo, S.; Koga, H.; Yagishita, K. Cross-sectional study on relationships between physical function and psychological readiness to return to sport after anterior cruciate ligament reconstruction. *BMC Sports Sci. Med. Rehabil.* **2022**, *14*, 97. [CrossRef] [PubMed]
14. Ueda, Y.; Matsushita, T.; Shibata, Y.; Takiguchi, K.; Ono, K.; Kida, A.; Ono, R.; Nagai, K.; Hoshino, Y.; Matsumoto, T.; et al. Association Between Meeting Return-to-Sport Criteria and Psychological Readiness to Return to Sport after Anterior Cruciate Ligament Reconstruction. *Orthop. J. Sports Med.* **2022**, *110*, 23259671221093985. [CrossRef] [PubMed]
15. King, E.; Richter, C.; Franklyn-Miller, A.; Franklyn-Miller, A.; Daniels, K.; Wadey, R.; Moran, R.; Strike, S. Whole-body biomechanical differences between limbs exist 9 months after ACL reconstruction across jump/landing tasks. *Scand J. Med. Sci. Sports* **2018**, *28*, 2567–2578. [CrossRef]
16. Thomeé, R.; Neeter, C.; Gustavsson, A.; Thomeé, P.; Augustsson, J.; Eriksson, B.; Karlsson, J. Variability in leg muscle power and hop performance after anterior cruciate ligament reconstruction. *Knee Surg. Sports Traumatol. Arthrosc.* **2012**, *20*, 1143–1151. [CrossRef]
17. Webster, K.E.; Feller, J.A. Evaluation of the Responsiveness of the Anterior Cruciate Ligament Return to Sport After Injury (ACL-RSI) Scale. *Orthop. J. Sports Med.* **2021**, *9*, 23259671211031240. [CrossRef]
18. Thiebat, G.; Cucchi, D.; Spreafico, A.; Muzzi, S.; Viganò, M.; Visconti, L.; Facchini, F.; de Girolamo, L. Italian version of the anterior cruciate ligament-return to sport after injury scale (IT ACL-RSI): Translation, cross-cultural adaptation, validation and ability to predict the return to sport at medium-term follow-up in a population of sport patients. *Knee. Surg. Sports Traumatol. Arthrosc.* **2022**, *30*, 270–279. [CrossRef]
19. McPherson, A.L.; Feller, J.A.; Hewett, T.E.; Webster, K.E. Psychological readiness to return to sport is associated with Second anterior cruciate ligament injuries. *Am. J. Sports Med.* **2019**, *47*, 857–862. [CrossRef]
20. Lysholm, J.; Gillquist, J. Evaluation of knee ligament surgery results with special emphasis on use of a scoring scale. *Am. J. Sports Med.* **1982**, *10*, 150–154. [CrossRef]
21. Padua, R.; Bondì, R.; Ceccarelli, E.; Bondì, L.; Romanini, E.; Zanoli, G.; Campi, S. Italian Version of the International Knee Documentation Committee Subjective Knee Form: Cross-Cultural Adaptation and Validation. *Arthroscopy* **2004**, *20*, 819–823. [CrossRef] [PubMed]
22. Tegner, Y.; Lysholm, J. Rating systems in the evaluation of knee ligament injuries. *Clin. Orthop. Relat. Res.* **1985**, *198*, 43–49. [CrossRef]
23. Gustavsson, A.; Neeter, C.; Thomeé, P.; Silbernagel, K.G.; Augustsson, J.; Thomeé, R.; Karlsson, J. A test battery for evaluating hop performance in patients with an ACL injury and patients who have undergone ACL reconstruction. *Knee Surg. Sports Traumatol. Arthrosc.* **2006**, *4*, 778–788. [CrossRef]
24. Ma, B.; Zhang, T.T.; Jia, Y.D.; Wang, H.; Zhu, X.Y.; Zhang, W.J.; Li, X.M.; Liu, H.B.; Xie, D. Characteristics of vertical drop jump to screen the anterior cruciate ligament injury. *Eur. Rev. Med. Pharmacol. Sci.* **2022**, *26*, 7395–7403. [PubMed]

25. Aizawa, J.; Hirohata, K.; Ohji, S.; Ohmi, T.; Koga, H.; Yagishita, K. Factors associated with psychological readiness to return to sports with cutting, pivoting, and jumplandings after primary ACL reconstruction. *Orthop. J. Sports Med.* **2020**, *8*, 2325967120964484. [PubMed]
26. Webster, K.E.; Nagelli, C.V.; Hewett, T.E.; Feller, J.A. Factors associated with psychological readiness to return to sport after anterior cruciate ligament reconstruction surgery. *Am. J. Sports Med.* **2018**, *46*, 1545–1550. [CrossRef] [PubMed]
27. Sadeqi, M.; Klouche, S.; Bohu, Y.; Herman, S.; Lefevre, N.; Gerometta, A. Progression of the psychological ACLRSI score and return to sport after anterior cruciate ligament reconstruction: A prospective 2-Year follow-up study from the French prospective anterior cruciate ligament reconstruction cohort study (FAST). *Orthop. J. Sports Med.* **2018**, *6*, 2325967118812819. [PubMed]
28. Senorski, E.H.; Svantesson, E.; Beischer, S.; Thomeé, C.; Thomeé, R.; Karlsson, J.; Samuelsson, K. Low 1-Year Return-to-Sport Rate After Anterior Cruciate Ligament Reconstruction Regardless of Patient and Surgical Factors A Prospective Cohort Study of 272 Patients. *Am. J. Sports Med.* **2018**, *46*, 1551–1558. [CrossRef] [PubMed]
29. Raizah, A.; Alhefzi, A.; Alshubruqi, A.A.M.; Hoban, M.A.M.A.; Ahmad, I.; Ahmad, F. Perceived Kinesiophobia and Its Association with Return to Sports Activity Following Anterior Cruciate Ligament Reconstruction Surgery: A Cross-Sectional Study. *Int. J. Environ. Res. Public Health* **2022**, *19*, 10776. [CrossRef]
30. Sánchez Romero, E.A.; Lim, T.; Alonso Pérez, J.L.; Castaldo, M.; Martínez Lozano, P.; Villafañe, J.H. Identifying Clinical and MRI Characteristics Associated with Quality of Life in Patients with Anterior Cruciate Ligament Injury: Prognostic Factors for Long-Term. *Int. J. Environ. Res. Public Health.* **2021**, *18*, 12845. [CrossRef]

Disclaimer/Publisher's Note: The statements, opinions and data contained in all publications are solely those of the individual author(s) and contributor(s) and not of MDPI and/or the editor(s). MDPI and/or the editor(s) disclaim responsibility for any injury to people or property resulting from any ideas, methods, instructions or products referred to in the content.

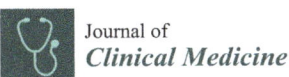

Article

Prophylactic Femoral Neck Fixation in an Osteoporosis Femur Model: A Novel Surgical Technique with Biomechanical Study

Kyeong-Hyeon Park [1], Joon-Woo Kim [1], Hee-Jun Kim [1], Dong-Hyun Kim [1], Jin-Han Lee [1], Won-Ki Hong [1] and Jong-Keon Oh [2]

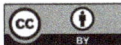

Citation: Park, K.-H.; Oh, C.-W.; Kim, J.-W.; Kim, H.-J.; Kim, D.-H.; Lee, J.-H.; Hong, W.-K.; Oh, J.-K. Prophylactic Femoral Neck Fixation in an Osteoporosis Femur Model: A Novel Surgical Technique with Biomechanical Study. *J. Clin. Med.* 2023, 12, 383. https://doi.org/10.3390/jcm12010383

Academic Editor: Yasuhiro Takeuchi

Received: 16 November 2022
Revised: 28 December 2022
Accepted: 1 January 2023
Published: 3 January 2023

Copyright: © 2023 by the authors. Licensee MDPI, Basel, Switzerland. This article is an open access article distributed under the terms and conditions of the Creative Commons Attribution (CC BY) license (https://creativecommons.org/licenses/by/4.0/).

[1] Department of Orthopedic Surgery, School of Medicine, Kyungpook National University, Kyungpook National University Hospital, Jung-gu, Daegu 41944, Republic of Korea
[2] Department of Orthopedic Surgery, School of Medicine, Korea University Guro Hospital, Seoul 10408, Republic of Korea
* Correspondence: cwoh@knu.ac.kr; Tel.: +82-53-420-5630

Abstract: Intramedullary nailing (IMN) is a popular treatment for elderly patients with femoral shaft fractures. Recently, prophylactic neck fixation has been increasingly used to prevent proximal femoral fractures during IMN. Therefore, this study aimed to investigate the biomechanical strength of prophylactic neck fixation in osteoporotic femoral fractures. An osteoporotic femur model was created to simulate the union of femoral shaft fractures with IMN. Two study groups comprising six specimens each were created for IMN with two standard proximal locking screws (SN group) and IMN with two reconstruction proximal locking screws (RN group). Axial loading was conducted to measure the stiffness, load-to-failure, and failure modes. There were no statistically significant differences in stiffness between the two groups. However, the load-to-failure in the RN group was significantly higher than that in the SN group ($p < 0.05$). Femoral neck fractures occurred in all specimens in the SN group. Five constructs in the RN group showed subtrochanteric fractures without femoral neck fractures. However, one construct was observed in both subtrochanteric and femoral neck fractures. Therefore, prophylactic neck fixation may be considered an alternative biomechanical solution to prevent proximal femoral fractures when performing IMN for osteoporotic femoral fractures.

Keywords: femur; nail; osteoporosis; prophylaxis

1. Introduction

Intramedullary (IM) nailing (IMN) is the preferred treatment method for femoral diaphyseal fractures in adults. As the elderly population increases, the selection of implants for the fixation of femoral shaft fractures in patients at a high risk of future fractures may be an essential process to ensure satisfactory outcomes. IM nail fixation is the standard treatment for femoral shaft fractures [1–3] and is increasing in popularity. However, late femoral neck and proximal peri-implant fractures have been reported after fixation of IMN without femoral neck protection of the femoral shaft fracture in elderly patients [4,5]. Additionally, the severity of osteoporosis is considered a significant risk factor for late hip fractures [4]. Thus, IMN can increase the risk of the femoral neck or proximal peri-implant fractures in elderly individuals with coexisting osteoporosis. This is because it can often be exacerbated by enforced postoperative immobility and a stress riser at the site of the proximal locking screw.

Many surgeons have recently selected a reconstruction nail (RN) with proximally directed interlocking screws to stabilize the femoral shaft and protect the femoral neck when treating femoral shaft fractures in elderly patients with osteoporosis. Several prior studies have investigated the role of prophylactic femoral neck fixation in diaphyseal femoral fractures [4–8] and have suggested that protecting the femoral neck during IM nail fixation of osteoporotic femoral shaft fractures may be effective in reducing late hip fractures [5–7].

In addition, a previous biomechanical study demonstrated that IM nail fixation with femoral neck protection can prevent femoral neck fractures [9]. However, it remains unclear whether the same biomechanical difference exists when IMN is performed in osteoporotic femoral models. This study investigated the biomechanical effect of prophylactic neck fixation on the proximal femur during IMN in an osteoporotic femur model.

2. Materials and Methods

Twelve synthetic osteoporotic femurs (Model 3503; Pacific Research Laboratories, Vashon, WA, USA) were used in this study. The femurs had a length of 455 mm, a 16 mm hollow canal, and an 18 mm inner cortical diameter. All synthetic femurs were stabilized with antegrade femoral nails (Expert A2FN, DePuy Synthes, Paoli, PA, USA) and divided into two groups according to femoral neck fixation. Six femurs were stabilized using two proximal standard interlocking screws (one oblique and one transverse screw) and two distal interlocking screws (SN group). The other six femurs were stabilized using two proximal reconstruction interlocking screws and two distal interlocking screws (RN group). A synthetic osteoporotic femur was used to simulate a femur with osteoporosis. Osteotomy was not performed after IM nail fixation in the femoral shaft fracture to ensure union.

2.1. Specimen Preparation

Each bone model was prepared according to the surgical techniques provided by the implant manufacturer. The nail was inserted at the tip of the greater trochanter (GT) in the anteroposterior (AP) view and parallel with the axial direction of the medullary cavity. The length of the nail was chosen such that its proximal end would meet the GT and its distal end could be placed in the supracondylar area of the distal femur. The length of the nail in the medullary cavity was 380 mm. Because the nail thickness was 10 mm, which was 2 mm less than the pre-measured thickness of the medullary cavity, the nail was inserted after reaming.

In the SN group, a 68 mm-long proximal locking screw was inserted in a 120° antegrade direction until it reached the cortex on the opposite side, for bicortical and firm fixation. Subsequently, a 50 mm-long locking screw was inserted into the static hole of the nail in the transverse direction. Both screws were 5.0 mm thick. In the RN group, two reconstruction screws were inserted and passed through the proximal and distal one-third of the femoral neck in the AP view and through the center of the lateral view. The screw length was chosen to match the distance to the subcortical bone of the femoral head. These hip screws had a thickness of 6.5 mm and lengths of 95 mm and 90 mm for the proximal and distal regions, respectively. After fixation of the proximal interlocking screws, two screws were inserted into the static hole in the distal nail region using a radiation amplifier in both groups. A single orthopedic surgeon performed all the procedures under fluoroscopic guidance to achieve a constant model for the biomechanical study. Proper implantation was confirmed on radiography after instrumentation (Figure 1).

2.2. Mechanical Loading

A load was applied to the head of the femur using a custom mold. Each potted femur was placed in a material testing machine (Electroplus E10000, Instron, Norwood, MA, USA) and held with custom fixation devices at 6° valgus to simulate anatomical positioning with weight bearing. The specimens were supported in the testing machine by a ball bearing to avoid uncontrolled torque or bending, as previously described by Cordey et al. [10]. Each distal femur was firmly held in a pre-shaped auto-polymerized acrylic resin (Vertex Dental, Zeist, Netherlands) until the lateral and medial condyles were in contact with the mold as it hardened. The mold aimed to evenly distribute the axial force applied during the testing process (Figure 2).

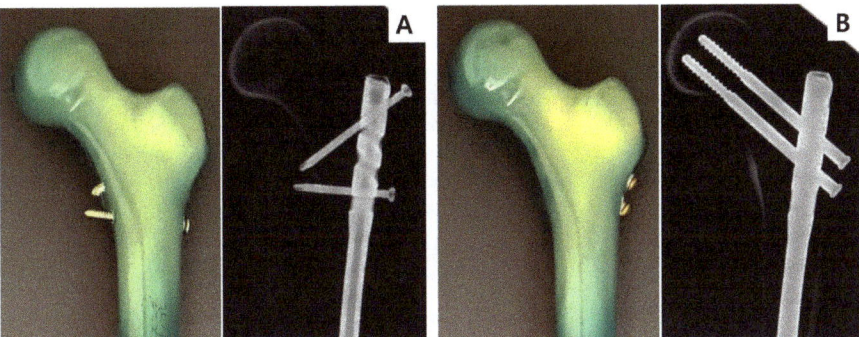

Figure 1. Two different constructs of the osteoporotic femur model with IMN and radiographs: (**A**) IMN with two standard proximal locking screws (SN group) and (**B**) IMN with two reconstruction proximal locking screws (RN group). IMN, intramedullary nailing.

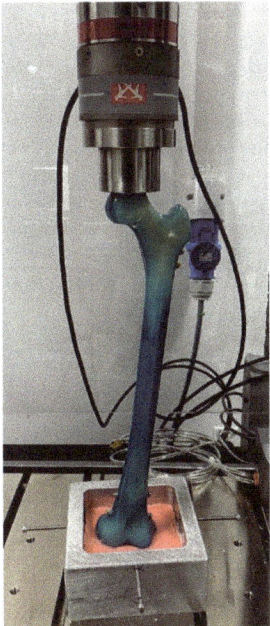

Figure 2. Experimental setup for measuring the stiffness and failure load after creating the osteoporotic femur models with different proximal interlocking screw constructs.

The experiments were designed to measure the structural stiffness, failure load, and failure mode of each proximal interlocking screw construct by applying axial compression. Before conducting the experiments, an axial preload of 100 N was applied to the servohydraulic testing machine and the femoral constructs to obtain stable results. The test was then performed by loading a 1500 N weight (twice the force applied to the femoral head of a 75 kg adult) at a velocity of 10 N/s in the direction of axial compression, as described by Grisell et al. [11]. This process was repeated five times, and the weight was loaded at 10 N/s on each femur until compressive failure. All constructs were ramped to failure by increasing the force to 10 N/s, and the load, displacement, and time data were collected at a sampling rate of 20 Hz. The axial displacements from the initial position to the preload and from the preload to the maximum load were continuously recorded using the crosshead motion sensor of the servohydraulic testing machine. The degree of displacement corresponding to the increase in axial load was determined for each femur. The stiffness of each femur was calculated as the slope of the elastic portion of the force versus displacement curve, and the mean value was considered. Failure was defined as screw breakage or fracture of a part of the construct, and the force applied to the femoral head at the time of failure was measured. If none of the aforementioned failure criteria were satisfied through direct observation, a sudden reduction in force, as revealed by the force versus displacement graph, was considered a failure [12].

2.3. Statistics

Independent sample *t*-tests were used to determine significant differences in stiffness, displacement, and mean failure load between screw constructs. A nonparametric alternative (Mann–Whitney U-test) was used if the hypothesis did not satisfy the parametric method. SPSS Statistics for Windows, Version 18.0 (SPSS Inc., Chicago, IL, USA), was used for statistical analyses, and statistical significance was set at $p < 0.05$.

3. Results

3.1. Stiffness and Load-to-Failure

There were no gross failures of any construct during or after the repeated cyclic load tests. The mean stiffness in the RN group was 8% higher than that in the SN group. However, there were no statistically significant differences between the two groups. The load-to-failure in the RN group was 25% higher than that in the SN group, and this difference was statistically significant. The descriptive data are presented in Table 1.

Table 1. Measurement results of construct stiffness under axial compressive load.

Construct	Axial Compressive Load	
	Stiffness (N/mm)	Load-to-Failure (N)
IM nail with standard interlocking screws (SN Group)	506 ± 37	2426 ± 163
IM nail with reconstruction interlocking screws (RN Group)	545 ± 57	3020 ± 103
p-value	0.31	<0.05

3.2. Mode of Failures

All constructs in the SN group failed similarly and resulted in basicervical femoral neck fractures from the GT nail entry hole through the proximal oblique interlocking screw (Figure 3A). In the RN group, the five constructs failed without any femoral neck fractures; two constructs sustained subtrochanteric fractures through the reconstruction screw hole without any femoral neck fractures, whereas three constructs sustained subtrochanteric fractures with a non-displaced fracture line that extended toward the GT entry holes. One construct was observed to have subtrochanteric and basicervical femoral neck fractures (Figure 3B).

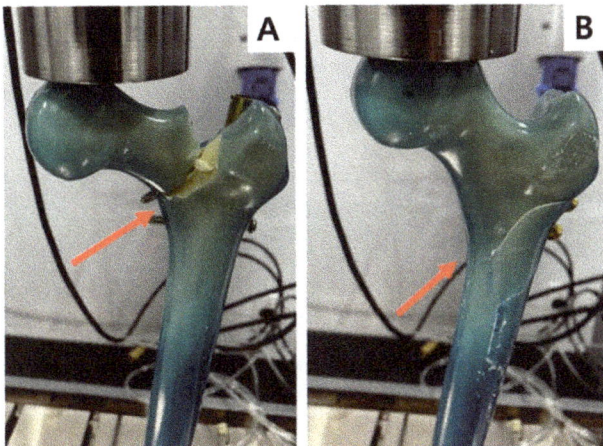

Figure 3. Failure modes after axial compressive loads. All constructs of group SN showed a basicervical femoral neck fracture from the GT nail entry hole through the proximal oblique interlocking screw (**A**). In the RN group reconstruction nail, five constructs exhibited a subtrochanteric fracture through the reconstruction screw hole, but without a femoral neck fracture (**B**). GT, greater trochanter. Red arrows point to the fracture lines.

4. Discussion

In this study, we evaluated the mechanical properties of prophylactic femoral neck fixation using reconstruction interlocking screws for IMN in an osteoporotic femur model. Our composite bone model simulated a healed femoral shaft fracture fixed with an IM nail for osteoporosis. Our findings revealed that the reconstruction interlocking constructs showed a higher load-to-failure and prevented delayed femoral neck fractures compared with the standard interlocking construct in an osteoporotic femur model.

Surgeons prefer prophylactic neck fixation for treating femoral fractures. Several authors have advocated prophylactic femoral neck fixation for all femoral shaft fractures because of concerns regarding iatrogenic or missed femoral neck fractures [6,7]. Patton et al. [4] reported late femoral neck fractures after IM nail fixation of femoral shaft fractures in elderly patients. Fourteen patients (2.7%) developed a proximal femoral fracture adjacent to an IM implant in their series. Among them, 11 fractures occurred within months to years. Most patients were > 60 years of age and had osteoporosis and low-energy injuries. Therefore, we suggest that prophylactic neck fixation during the construction of osteoporotic femoral shaft fractures with a reconstruction nail is necessary. Bögl et al. [5] reviewed 897 patients treated for low-energy diaphyseal femoral fractures in Sweden. In their study, 640 patients were treated with IM nails with femoral neck fixation, whereas 257 patients were treated without femoral neck protection. The authors found a fivefold decrease in the risk of reoperation for peri-implant fractures and half the risk of major reoperation when treated with femoral neck fixation. Our study also demonstrated biomechanically that prophylactic neck fixation could effectively prevent femoral neck fractures after IMN for osteoporotic femoral shaft fractures.

Few biomechanical studies have been conducted on prophylactic neck fixation. Previous biomechanical studies using piriformis entry nails have reported that the load-to-failure was similar, regardless of femoral neck protection [13]. They postulated that this may have resulted from a large entry hole through the piriformis fossa, which created a significant bone defect at the base of the femoral neck. Another study using a GT entry nail with neck protection showed a higher load-to-failure than a piriformis entry nail, similar to that of an intact femur [9]. In the present study, higher load-to-failure values were observed in the RN group. This is the result of the difference between the nail entry portal and composite bone used. For osteoporotic femoral shaft treatment, GT entry nail and prophylactic neck fixation may be considered appropriate.

The location of the entry site contributes to the strength of the femoral neck during fixation. In a cadaveric study, Miller et al. [14] showed that the entry site of the piriformis fossa could significantly weaken the neck. All the specimens in their study sustained basicervical fracture patterns under mechanical loading. Strand et al. [15] conducted a cadaveric study comparing entry portals at either the piriformis fossa or the GT of the cadaver. All femurs of the piriformis fossa entry portals sustained basicervical fractures at the entry site. The piriformis fossa group showed a lower load-to-failure than the GT group. As elderly patients with osteoporosis have a lower bone density around the femoral neck, the piriformis entry portal may pose a higher risk of femoral neck fractures in these patients. When performing nailing for femoral fractures, especially in elderly patients, avoiding the piriformis entry portal is recommended. Therefore, our experimental procedure was conducted using the trochanter entry portal.

Synthetic femurs have been widely used and accepted as a substitute for cadaveric specimens in biomechanics. Recently, a new osteoporotic synthetic femur has been introduced by the increasing osteoporosis population. The wall thickness and bone density were reduced to simulate osteoporotic bone. In biomechanical studies, the osteoporotic synthetic bone shows similar axial loading results compared with the osteoporotic bone [16].

Our study had several limitations. First, this was a biomechanical study using synthetic femur models and, thus, may not accurately represent human bone mechanics, especially in elderly patients. However, synthetic bone provides several advantages over cadaveric bone; thus, it is preferred in biomechanical studies [12,17]. Furthermore, synthetic bones can provide standard sizes and properties between specimens and guarantee implantation techniques' reproducibility. In addition, cadaveric specimens of varying dimensions, ages, and bone densities were excluded. Moreover, our approach is meaningful because we used a newly developed synthetic osteoporotic bone biomechanically similar to an osteoporotic cadaveric femur [16].

Second, the axial load provided by a mechanical testing machine may not accurately mimic the physiological load or vector experienced during a standard ground-level fall. We assumed that femur neck fracture is a result of axial load through the mechanical axis of the femur. We decided to use this assumption to enhance reproducibility, with the thought that weight bearing goes through the mechanical axis from a functional perspective. Other forces we did not simulate can cause femur neck fractures. However, the testing model used in this study has been validated and previously utilized in multiple biomechanical studies. Consequently, this is an appropriate and applicable method for isolating the strength of the proximal femur.

Third, we only tested load-to-failure rather than cyclic loading. Failure loading simulates a fall or other trauma. Moreover, some clinical reports had either no or minimal trauma due to the mechanism of the fracture, implying that femur neck fracture may be due to repetitive loading, leading to a stress fracture. However, our goal was to investigate the protection the fixation construct provides against a catastrophic event such as a fall.

Finally, this study was conducted only with an osteoporotic bone model, so the effect of prophylactic neck fixation is specific to the osteoporotic femur. Additional samples and comparison studies with non-osteoporotic bone may have provided a more accurate representation of the load-to-failure of the femur models.

5. Conclusions

In summary, the results of this biomechanical study showed that femoral nailing with two reconstruction screws resulted in a higher load-to-failure than femoral nailing with standard screws in an osteoporotic femoral model. Clinically, it may be assumed that IM nail fixation using reconstructive screws could prevent femoral neck fractures in patients with osteoporosis.

Author Contributions: Conceptualization, K.-H.P. and C.-W.O.; methodology, J.-W.K. and H.-J.K.; validation, W.-K.H.; formal analysis, K.-H.P.; investigation, K.-H.P. and J.-H.L.; data curation, D.-H.K. and H.-J.K.; writing—original draft preparation, K.-H.P.; writing—review, and editing, C.-W.O. and J.-K.O.; visualization, K.-H.P.; supervision, C.-W.O. All authors have read and agreed to the published version of the manuscript.

Funding: This work was supported by the National Research Foundation of Korea (NRF) grant funded by the Korea government (MSIT) (No. 2020R1G1A1009982).

Institutional Review Board Statement: Not applicable.

Informed Consent Statement: Not applicable.

Data Availability Statement: Source data may be shared upon reasonable request to the corresponding author.

Conflicts of Interest: The authors declare no conflict of interest.

References

1. Neumann, M.V.; Südkamp, N.P.; Strohm, P.C. Management of femoral shaft fractures. *Acta Chir. Orthop. Traumatol. Cech.* **2015**, *82*, 22–32. [PubMed]
2. Elbarbary, A.N.; Hassen, S.; Badr, I.T. Outcome of intramedullary nail for fixation of osteoporotic femoral shaft fractures in the elderly above 60. *Injury* **2021**, *52*, 602–605. [CrossRef] [PubMed]
3. Tano, A.; Oh, Y.; Fukushima, K.; Kurosa, Y.; Wakabayashi, Y.; Fujita, K.; Yoshii, T.; Okawa, A. Potential bone fragility of mid-shaft atypical femoral fracture: Biomechanical analysis by a CT-based nonlinear finite element method. *Injury* **2019**, *50*, 1876–1882. [CrossRef] [PubMed]
4. Patton, J.T.; Cook, R.E.; Adams, C.I.; Robinson, C.M. Late fracture of the hip after reamed intramedullary nailing of the femur. *J. Bone Jt. Surg. Br.* **2000**, *82*, 967–971. [CrossRef] [PubMed]
5. Bögl, H.P.; Zdolsek, G.; Michaëlsson, K.; Höijer, J.; Schilcher, J. Reduced Risk of Reoperation Using Intramedullary Nailing with Femoral Neck Protection in Low-Energy Femoral Shaft Fractures. *J. Bone Jt. Surg. Am.* **2020**, *102*, 1486–1494. [CrossRef] [PubMed]
6. Collinge, C.; Liporace, F.; Koval, K.; Gilbert, G.T. Cephalomedullary screws as the standard proximal locking screws for nailing femoral shaft fractures. *J. Orthop. Trauma* **2010**, *24*, 717–722. [CrossRef] [PubMed]
7. Faucett, S.C.; Collinge, C.A.; Koval, K.J. Is reconstruction nailing of all femoral shaft fractures cost effective? A decision analysis. *J. Orthop. Trauma* **2012**, *26*, 624–632. [CrossRef] [PubMed]
8. Moon, B.; Lin, P.; Satcher, R.; Bird, J.; Lewis, V. Intramedullary nailing of femoral diaphyseal metastases: Is it necessary to protect the femoral neck? *Clin. Orthop.* **2015**, *473*, 1499–1502. [CrossRef] [PubMed]
9. Shieh, A.K.; Bravin, D.A.; Shelton, T.J.; Garcia-Nolen, T.C.; Lee, M.A.; Eastman, J.G. A Biomechanical Comparison of Trochanteric Versus Piriformis Reconstruction Nails for Femoral Neck Fracture Prophylaxis. *J. Orthop. Trauma* **2021**, *35*, e293–e297. [CrossRef] [PubMed]
10. Cordey, J.; Borgeaud, M.; Frankle, M.; Harder, Y.; Martinet, O. Loading model for the human femur taking the tension band effect of the ilio-tibial tract into account. *Injury* **1999**, *30* (Suppl. S1), A26–A30. [CrossRef] [PubMed]
11. Grisell, M.; Moed, B.R.; Bledsoe, J.G. A biomechanical comparison of trochanteric nail proximal screw configurations in a subtrochanteric fracture model. *J. Orthop. Trauma* **2010**, *24*, 359–363. [CrossRef] [PubMed]
12. Kim, J.W.; Oh, C.W.; Byun, Y.S.; Oh, J.K.; Kim, H.J.; Min, W.K.; Park, S.K.; Park, B.C. A biomechanical analysis of locking plate fixation with minimally invasive plate osteosynthesis in a subtrochanteric fracture model. *J. Trauma* **2011**, *70*, E19–E23. [CrossRef] [PubMed]
13. Shieh, A.K.; Refaat, M.; Heyrani, N.; Garcia-Nolen, T.C.; Lee, M.A.; Eastman, J.G. Are piriformis reconstruction implants ideal for prophylactic femoral neck fixation? *Injury* **2019**, *50*, 703–707. [CrossRef] [PubMed]
14. Miller, S.D.; Burkart, B.; Damson, E.; Shrive, N.; Bray, R.C. The effect of the entry hole for an intramedullary nail on the strength of the proximal femur. *J. Bone Jt. Surg. Br.* **1993**, *75*, 202–206. [CrossRef] [PubMed]
15. Strand, R.M.; Mølster, A.O.; Engesaeter, L.B.; Gjerdet, N.R.; Orner, T. Mechanical effects of different localization of the point of entry in femoral nailing. *Arch. Orthop. Trauma Surg.* **1998**, *117*, 35–38. [CrossRef] [PubMed]
16. Gluek, C.; Zdero, R.; Quenneville, C.E. Evaluating the mechanical response of novel synthetic femurs for representing osteoporotic bone. *J. Biomech.* **2020**, *111*, 110018. [CrossRef] [PubMed]
17. Park, K.-H.; Oh, C.-W.; Park, I.-H.; Kim, J.-W.; Lee, J.-H.; Kim, H.-J. Additional fixation of medial plate over the unstable lateral locked plating of distal femur fractures: A biomechanical study. *Injury* **2019**, *50*, 1593–1598. [CrossRef] [PubMed]

Disclaimer/Publisher's Note: The statements, opinions and data contained in all publications are solely those of the individual author(s) and contributor(s) and not of MDPI and/or the editor(s). MDPI and/or the editor(s) disclaim responsibility for any injury to people or property resulting from any ideas, methods, instructions or products referred to in the content.

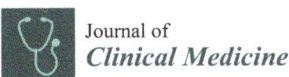

Article

The Association between the Hematocrit at Admission and Preoperative Deep Venous Thrombosis in Hip Fractures in Older People: A Retrospective Analysis

Dong-Yang Li [1], Dong-Xing Lu [1], Ting Yan [2], Kai-Yuan Zhang [2], Bin-Fei Zhang [3,*] and Yu-Min Zhang [3,*]

1. Department of Orthopedic Trauma, Honghui Hospital, Xi'an Jiaotong University, Xi'an 710054, China
2. Department of Ultrasound Medicine, Honghui Hospital, Xi'an Jiaotong University, Xi'an 710054, China
3. Department of Joint Surgery, Honghui Hospital, Xi'an Jiaotong University, Xi'an 710054, China
* Correspondence: zhangbf07@gmail.com (B.-F.Z.); zym2666@126.com (Y.-M.Z.)

Abstract: Hematocrit, a commonly used hematological indicator, is a simple and easily applicable test. As a marker of anisocytosis and anemia, it indicates the percentage of blood cells per unit volume of whole blood. This study aimed to evaluate the association between the level of the hematocrit at admission and preoperative deep vein thrombosis (DVT) in hip fractures of older people. We collected the demographic and clinical characteristics of patients with geriatric hip fractures between 1 January 2015, and 30 September 2019, at the largest trauma center in northwestern China. Doppler ultrasonography was used to diagnose DVT. The correlation between hematocrit levels at admission and preoperative DVT was assessed using linear and nonlinear multivariate logistic regression, according to the adjusted model. All analyzes were performed using EmpowerStats and R software. In total, 1840 patients were included in this study, of which 587 patients (32%) had preoperative DVT. The mean hematocrit level was 34.44 ± 5.64 vol%. Linear multivariate logistic regression models showed that admission hematocrit levels were associated with preoperative DVT (OR = 0.97, 95% CI: 0.95–0.99; $p = 0.0019$) after adjustment for confounding factors. However, the linear association was unstable, and nonlinearity was identified. An admission hematocrit level of 33.5 vol% was an inflection point for the prediction. Admission hematocrit levels <33.5 vol% were not associated with preoperative DVT (OR = 1.00, 95% CI: 0.97–1.04, $p = 0.8230$), whereas admission hematocrit levels >33.5 vol% were associated with preoperative DVT (OR = 0.94, 95% CI: 25 0.91–0.97, $p = 0.0006$). Hematocrit levels at admission were nonlinearly associated with preoperative DVT, and hematocrit at admission was a risk factor for preoperative DVT. However, the severity of a low hematocrit was not associated with preoperative DVT when the hematocrit was <33.5 vol%.

Keywords: hematocrit; hip fracture; DVT; logistic regression; retrospective

Citation: Li, D.-Y.; Lu, D.-X.; Yan, T.; Zhang, K.-Y.; Zhang, B.-F.; Zhang, Y.-M. The Association between the Hematocrit at Admission and Preoperative Deep Venous Thrombosis in Hip Fractures in Older People: A Retrospective Analysis. *J. Clin. Med.* **2023**, *12*, 353. https://doi.org/10.3390/jcm12010353

Academic Editor: Heinrich Resch

Received: 6 December 2022
Revised: 28 December 2022
Accepted: 29 December 2022
Published: 2 January 2023

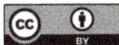

Copyright: © 2023 by the authors. Licensee MDPI, Basel, Switzerland. This article is an open access article distributed under the terms and conditions of the Creative Commons Attribution (CC BY) license (https://creativecommons.org/licenses/by/4.0/).

1. Introduction

As the main type of osteoporotic fracture, hip fractures have a high incidence in the older population [1]. The number of hip fractures worldwide is estimated to reach 4.5 million by 2050 [2]. With the aging population and longer life expectancy, patients with hip fractures are a major challenge for the healthcare system and society due to poor prognosis [3–5]. Patients with hip fractures often have other diseases and are in poor physical condition. Therefore, older adults are at risk for prolonged bed rest after hip fractures.

Kaperonis et al. found that 5-day bed rest in a normal person results in sluggish blood flow, increased red blood cell aggregation, and increased blood viscosity, which can induce deep vein thrombosis (DVT) [6]. DVT is common in older adults with hip fractures due to trauma, immobilization, advanced age, and comorbidities [7,8]. The reported prevalence of perioperative DVT after hip fracture ranges from 11.1 to 29.4% [9,10].

For patients at high risk of thrombosis, proactive measures should be taken in time to prevent and treat DVT. Otherwise, it can lead to chronic pain, and secondary varicose, even fatal, pulmonary embolism (PE) can occur, which seriously affects the quality of life and increases the hospitalization costs [11,12]. There has been considerable research on the prevention of DVT, but optimal preventive measures have not been established. Rivaroxaban or low-molecular-weight heparin (LMWH) is a treatment for DVT prophylaxis [13,14]. However, it has not been particularly effective. The incidence of DVT is still 20–30% [10,15]. Therefore, it is necessary to analyze in depth the risk factors for perioperative DVT, which may help prevent the further development of this complication.

The hematocrit is a commonly used hematological indicator as a marker for anisocytosis and anemia, and indicates the percentage of red blood cells per unit volume of whole blood [16]. It is one of the main determinants of blood viscosity, and an increased hematocrit is associated with increased blood viscosity, decreased venous return, and increased exposure of endothelial cells to platelets and coagulation factors [17]. Therefore, subjects with Hct levels above the normal range are theoretically susceptible to DVT. Previous studies have shown a correlation between Hct level and DVT. However, the relationship between hematocrit and DVT is not sufficiently detailed and remains controversial [18–20]. Data from previous studies were based on the general population rather than on patients with fractures. Regarding hip fractures in older adults, evidence on the relationship between the hematocrit level at admission and preoperative DVT is lacking. Therefore, it is necessary to build a reliable model to understand the association between Hct levels at admission and DVT or to predict the prognosis.

This study aimed to evaluate the association between the level of the hematocrit at admission and preoperative DVT in older adults with hip fractures. We hypothesized that there is a linear or nonlinear association between hematocrit level at admission and preoperative DVT, which would explain the effect of hematocrit level at admission on preoperative DVT and provide a target for prevention.

2. Materials and Methods

2.1. Ethics Statement

We recruited older adults with a hip fracture between 1 January 2015, and 30 September 2019, at the largest trauma center in Northwest China.

The Ethics Committee of our hospital (No. 202201009) approved this retrospective study. All human procedures were performed in accordance with the Declaration of Helsinki of 1964 and its subsequent amendments. The study was conducted according to the STROCSS 2021 guidelines [21].

2.2. Inclusion and Exclusion Criteria

The demographic and clinical data of the patients were obtained from their original medical records. The inclusion criteria were as follows: (1) age ≥65 years; (2) diagnosis by X-ray or computed tomography of femoral neck or intertrochanteric or subtrochanteric fracture; and (3) patients receiving surgical or conservative treatment in the hospital. The exclusion criteria were as follows: patients for whom clinical data in the hospital were unavailable.

2.3. Hospital Treatment

The patients were examined using blood tests and ultrasonography to prepare for surgery. Prophylaxis for deep vein thrombosis was initiated at admission. A mechanical pressure pump (20 min, twice daily) was used to promote blood reflux. Furthermore, for patients without contraindications, LMWH was subcutaneously injected according to guidelines to prevent DVT. Anticoagulant therapy was discontinued 12 h before the operation and resumed 24 h after the operation. Blood samples were collected at the time of admission (2 h after admission).

2.4. DVT Diagnosis

According to Chinese guidelines for the prevention of venous thromboembolism in orthopedic surgery, color Doppler ultrasound was used to detect DVT. Vascular ultrasonography was performed using a bedside machine by three trained operators. The diagnostic criterion for fresh thrombosis was the presence of a constant intraluminal filling defect [22], as shown in Figure 1. Anticoagulation regimens were guided by hospital consultations during vascular surgery. If required, an inferior vena cava filter was used to prevent fatal pulmonary embolism.

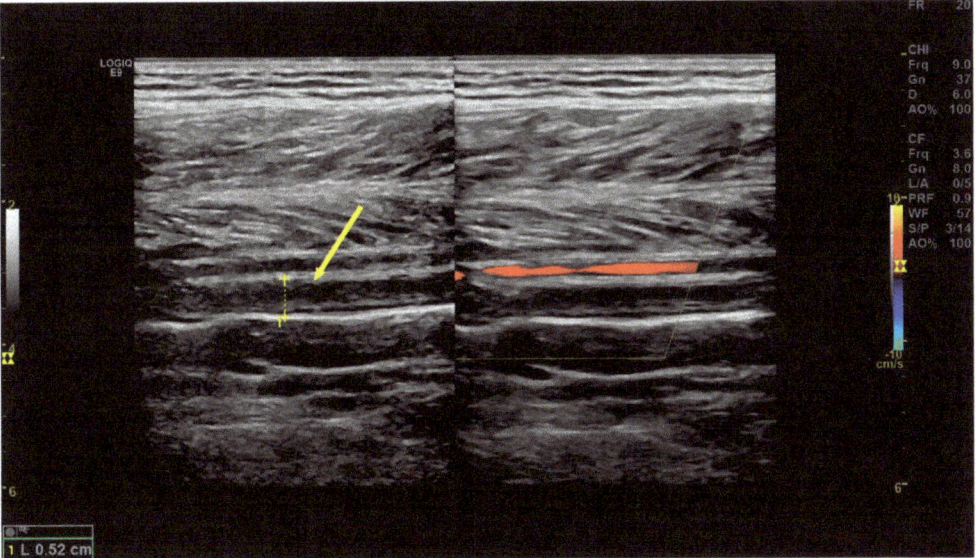

Figure 1. DVT in Doppler ultrasonography (yellow arrow).

2.5. Endpoint Events

The endpoint event in this study was preoperative DVT.

2.6. Variables

In this study, the following variables were collected: hematocrit level, age, sex, occupation, history of allergy, injury mechanism, fracture classification, hypertension, diabetes, coronary heart disease, arrhythmia, hemorrhagic stroke, ischemic stroke, cancer, associated injuries, dementia, chronic obstructive pulmonary disease (COPD), hepatitis, gastritis, age–adjusted Charlson comorbidity index (aCCI), and time from injury to admission.

The dependent variable was preoperative DVT, and the independent variable was the level of the hematocrit. Other variables were confounding factors.

2.7. Statistics Analysis

Descriptive statistical analyzes were performed using standard reporting methods. Continuous variables are reported as mean ± standard deviation (normally distributed data) or median (interquartile range) (nonnormally distributed data). Categorical variables were reported as percentages. Chi–square (categorical variables), one–way ANOVA (normal distribution), or Kruskal–Wallis H tests (skewed distribution) were used to detect differences among different levels of the hematocrit at admission.

We analyzed the association between Hct level and preoperative DVT. Univariate and multivariate binary logistic regression models were used to test the association between Hct levels and preoperative DVT using three distinct models. Model 1: No covariates are adjusted. Model 2 was a minimally adjusted model, adjusted only for sociodemographic covariates. Model 3 was fully adjusted for all covariates. We performed a sensitivity analysis to verify the robustness of the results. We converted admission hematocrit into a categorical variable according to the quintiles, calculated p for the trend to verify the results of admission hematocrit as a continuous variable, and examined the possibility of nonlinearity (Q1–Q5 groups).

To account for the nonlinear relationship between hematocrit and preoperative DVT, we also used a generalized additive model and smooth curve fitting (penalized spline method) to address nonlinearity. If nonlinearity was detected, we first calculated the inflection point using a recursive algorithm and then constructed a two-piece logistic proportional hazard regression model for each side of the inflection point.

All analyzes were performed using the statistical software packages R (http://www.R-project.org, R Foundation, Vienna, Austria) (accessed on 25 September 2022) and Empower-Stats (http://www.empowerstats.com, X&Y Solutions Inc., Boston, MA, USA) (accessed on 25 September 2022). Statistical significance was established by a two-sided p-value, where $p < 0.05$ (two-sided) was considered to be statistically significant.

3. Results

3.1. Patient Characteristics

Of the 1881 participants with hip fractures between January 2015 and September 2019, 48 patients were excluded from this study due to missing HCT data at admission. A total of 1840 patients met the study criteria and were enrolled in our study. A flowchart is shown in Figure 2. Hematocrit levels were divided into five groups. The average admission hematocrit of all patients was 34.44 ± 5.64 vol% (Q1 group: 25.35 ± 2.96 vol%, Q2 group: 30.62 ± 1.08 vol%, Q3 group: 33.75 ± 0.83 vol%, Q4 group: 36.61 ± 0.88 vol%, and Q5 group: 41.29 ± 2.67 vol%). A total of 587 patients (32%) had preoperative DVT ((Q1 group: 95 (33.69%); Q2 group: 120 (36.70%); Q3 group: 135 (37.92%); Q4 group: 125 (30.19%); and Q5 group: 112 (24.30%)). Eight patients had pulmonary embolism, and two died after the operation due to coronary heart disease (CHD).

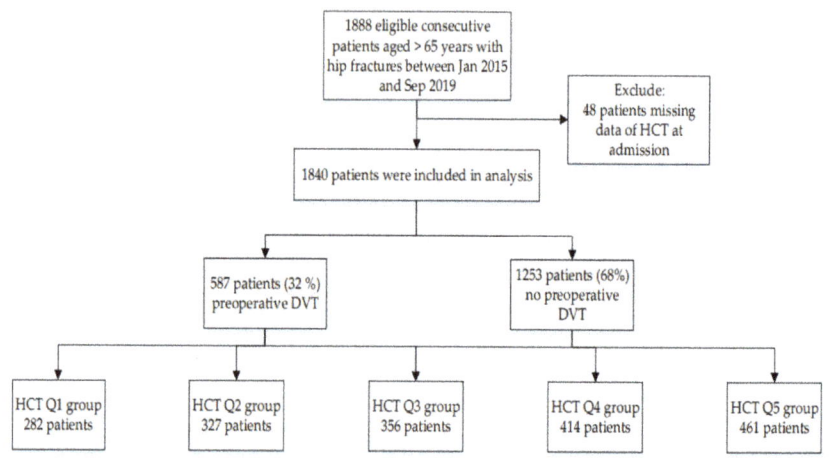

Figure 2. Study flow diagram.

Table 1 lists the demographic and clinical characteristics of all 1840 patients, including comorbidities, factors associated with injuries, and hematocrit levels at admission.

Table 1. The demographic and clinical characteristics of the patients (N = 1840).

Hematocrit Quintiles	Q1 (n = 282)	Q2 (n = 327)	Q3 (n = 356)	Q4 (n = 414)	Q5 (n = 461)	p-Value	p-Value *
Age (year)	82.61 ± 6.32	80.53 ± 6.90	79.62 ± 6.30	78.66 ± 6.57	77.14 ± 6.98	<0.001	<0.001
Sex						<0.001	-
Male	55 (19.50%)	89 (27.22%)	94 (26.40%)	109 (26.33%)	211 (45.77%)		
Female	227 (80.50%)	238 (72.78%)	262 (73.60%)	305 (73.67%)	250 (54.23%)		
Injury mechanism						0.527	-
Falling	272 (96.45%)	317 (96.94%)	339 (95.22%)	404 (97.58%)	441 (95.66%)		
Traffic accident	7 (2.48%)	7 (2.14%)	14 (3.93%)	10 (2.42%)	15 (3.25%)		
Other	3 (1.06%)	3 (0.92%)	3 (0.84%)	0 (0.00%)	5 (1.08%)		
Fracture classification						<0.001	-
Intertrochanteric fracture	228 (80.85%)	261 (79.82%)	236 (66.29%)	199 (48.07%)	182 (39.48%)		
Femoral neck fracture	45 (15.96%)	59 (18.04%)	113 (31.74%)	208 (50.24%)	276 (59.87%)		
Subtrochanteric fracture	9 (3.19%)	7 (2.14%)	7 (1.97%)	7 (1.69%)	3 (0.65%)		
Hypertension	123 (43.62%)	160 (48.93%)	184 (51.69%)	203 (49.03%)	254 (55.10%)	0.039	-
Diabetes	45 (15.96%)	60 (18.35%)	82 (23.03%)	82 (19.81%)	98 (21.26%)	0.202	-
CHD	142 (50.35%)	163 (49.85%)	193 (54.21%)	198 (47.83%)	254 (55.10%)	0.187	-
Arrhythmia	98 (34.75%)	97 (29.66%)	107 (30.06%)	113 (27.29%)	168 (36.44%)	0.029	-
Hemorrhagic stroke	5 (1.77%)	6 (1.83%)	6 (1.69%)	5 (1.21%)	10 (2.17%)	0.877	-
Ischemic stroke	82 (29.08%)	104 (31.80%)	111 (31.18%)	114 (27.54%)	169 (36.66%)	0.05	-
Cancer	7 (2.48%)	13 (3.98%)	9 (2.53%)	11 (2.66%)	8 (1.74%)	0.431	-
Dementia	20 (7.09%)	8 (2.45%)	10 (2.81%)	18 (4.35%)	15 (3.25%)	0.022	-
Multiple injuries	36 (12.77%)	31 (9.48%)	23 (6.46%)	23 (5.56%)	18 (3.90%)	<0.001	-
COPD	17 (6.03%)	18 (5.50%)	21 (5.90%)	19 (4.59%)	31 (6.72%)	0.75	-
Hepatitis	15 (5.32%)	6 (1.83%)	10 (2.81%)	11 (2.66%)	13 (2.82%)	0.135	-
Gastritis	6 (2.13%)	4 (1.22%)	9 (2.53%)	5 (1.21%)	3 (0.65%)	0.194	-
Time to admission (h)	71.83 ± 122.56	80.71 ± 159.64	86.29 ± 263.66	108.05 ± 407.03	70.30 ± 172.10	0.22	<0.001
aCCI	4.49 ± 0.99	4.28 ± 1.05	4.27 ± 1.16	4.11 ± 1.17	4.05 ± 1.07	<0.001	<0.001
Hematocrit	25.35 ± 2.96 (11.90–28.50)	30.62 ± 1.08 (28.60–32.20)	33.75 ± 0.83 (32.30–35.10)	36.61 ± 0.88 (35.20–38.20)	41.29 ± 2.67 (38.30–54.20)	<0.001	<0.001
DVT	95 (33.69%)	120 (36.70%)	135 (37.92%)	125 (30.19%)	112 (24.30%)	<0.001	-

Mean ± SD/N (%). p-value *: For continuous variables, we used the Kruskal–Wallis rank-sum test, and Fisher's exact probability test was used for count variables with a theoretical number <10.

3.2. Univariate Analysis

To identify possible confounders and the relationship between admission hematocrit level and preoperative DVT, we performed a univariate analysis (Table 2). According to the criteria of $p < 0.1$, the following variables were considered in the multivariate logistic regression: sex, dementia, and multiple injuries.

Table 2. Effects of factors on preoperative DVT measured by univariate analysis (N = 1840).

	Statistics	OR (95% CI)	p-Value
Age (year)	79.40 ± 6.88	1.00 (0.99, 1.02)	0.7005
Sex			
Male	558 (30.33%)	1	
Female	1282 (69.67%)	1.26 (1.01, 1.56)	0.0388
Injury mechanism			
Falling	1773 (96.36%)	1	
Traffic accident	53 (2.88%)	1.11 (0.62, 1.98)	0.7206
Other	14 (0.76%)	2.88 (0.99, 8.34)	0.0511
Fracture classification			
Intertrochanteric fracture	1106 (60.11%)	1	
Femoral neck fracture	701 (38.10%)	0.68 (0.56, 0.84)	0.0004
Subtrochanteric fracture	33 (1.79%)	1.77 (0.88, 3.54)	0.1069
Time to admission (h)	83.97 ± 255.05	1.00 (1.00, 1.00)	0.2535
Hypertension			
No	916 (49.78%)	1	
Yes	924 (50.22%)	1.13 (0.93, 1.38)	0.2215
Diabetes			
No	1473 (80.05%)	1	
Yes	367 (19.95%)	0.95 (0.74, 1.22)	0.6998
CHD			
No	890 (48.37%)	1	
Yes	950 (51.63%)	1.07 (0.88, 1.30)	0.488
Arrhythmia			
No	1257 (68.32%)	1	
Yes	583 (31.68%)	1.07 (0.87, 1.32)	0.5182
Hemorrhagic stroke			
No	1808 (98.26%)	1	
Yes	32 (1.74%)	1.68 (0.83, 3.39)	0.1512
Ischemic stroke			
No	1260 (68.48%)	1	
Yes	580 (31.52%)	0.86 (0.69, 1.06)	0.1608
Cancer			
No	1792 (97.39%)	1	
Yes	48 (2.61%)	1.18 (0.65, 2.14)	0.5969
Dementia			
No	1769 (96.14%)	1	
Yes	71 (3.86%)	1.59 (0.98, 2.58)	0.0583

Table 2. Cont.

	Statistics	OR (95% CI)	*p*-Value
Multiple injuries			
No	1709 (92.88%)	1	
Yes	131 (7.12%)	1.60 (1.12, 2.30)	0.0108
COPD			
No	1734 (94.24%)	1	
Yes	106 (5.76%)	0.88 (0.57, 1.35)	0.5457
Hepatitis			
No	1785 (97.01%)	1	
Yes	55 (2.99%)	0.65 (0.35, 1.23)	0.1849
Gastritis			
No	1813 (98.53%)	1	
Yes	27 (1.47%)	0.48 (0.18, 1.28)	0.1413
aCCI	4.21 ± 1.10	0.99 (0.91, 1.09)	0.8784
Hematocrit	34.44 ± 5.64	0.97 (0.95, 0.98)	0.0002

3.3. Multivariate Analysis between Admission Hematocrit Level and Preoperative DVT

We used three models (Table 3) to correlate hematocrit levels and preoperative DVT. When the hematocrit level was a continuous variable, linear regression was observed. The fully adjusted model showed a preoperative decrease in the risk of DVT of 3% (OR = 0.97, 95% CI: 0.95–0.99, p = 0.0019) when hematocrit levels increased by 1% after controlling for confounders. When hematocrit levels were used as a categorical variable, we found statistically significant differences in the hematocrit level groups of the three models ($p < 0.05$). Compared with the hematocrit Q1 group, the hematocrit Q5 group could decrease the risk of preoperative DVT by 31% (OR = 0.69, 95% CI: 0.50–0.97, p = 0.0304). However, there were no statistically significant differences among the Q2–Q4 hematocrit groups and the Q1 group. In addition, the p for the trend showed $p < 0.05$ in the three models. This instability indicates a nonlinear correlation.

Table 3. Multivariate results by logistic regression (N = 1840).

Exposure	Non-Adjusted Model	Minimally-Adjusted Model	Fully-Adjusted Model
Hematocrit	0.97 (0.95, 0.98) 0.0002	0.97 (0.95, 0.99) 0.0006	0.97 (0.95, 0.99) 0.0019
Hematocrit quintiles			
Q1	1	1	1
Q2	1.14 (0.82, 1.59) 0.4385	1.15 (0.83, 1.61) 0.3996	1.20 (0.85, 1.68) 0.2943
Q3	1.20 (0.87, 1.67) 0.2689	1.22 (0.88, 1.69) 0.2431	1.27 (0.92, 1.77) 0.1494
Q4	0.85 (0.62, 1.18) 0.3305	0.86 (0.62, 1.19) 0.3626	0.90 (0.65, 1.24) 0.5175
Q5	0.63 (0.46, 0.88) 0.0058	0.66 (0.47, 0.91) 0.0129	0.69 (0.50, 0.97) 0.0304
P for trend	0.0002	0.0007	0.002

Data in table: OR (95% CI), *p*-value. Outcome variable: preoperative DVT. Exposure variable: hematocrit level at admission. Minimally-adjusted model: adjust for sex. Fully-adjusted model: adjust for sex, dementia, and multiple injuries.

3.4. Curve Fitting and Analysis of Threshold Effect

As shown in Figure 3, after adjusting for confounders, we fit a curve to explain the association between Hct levels at admission and preoperative DVT. We compared two fitting models to explain this association (Table 4). Interestingly, an inflection point was observed. Admission hematocrit levels of >33.5 vol% were associated with preoperative DVT (OR = 0.94, 95% CI: 0.91–0.97, p = 0.0006). At admission hematocrit levels of <33.5 vol%, there was no statistically significant correlation between preoperative DVT and admission hematocrit levels (OR = 0.94, 95% CI: 0.91–0.97, p = 0.0006).

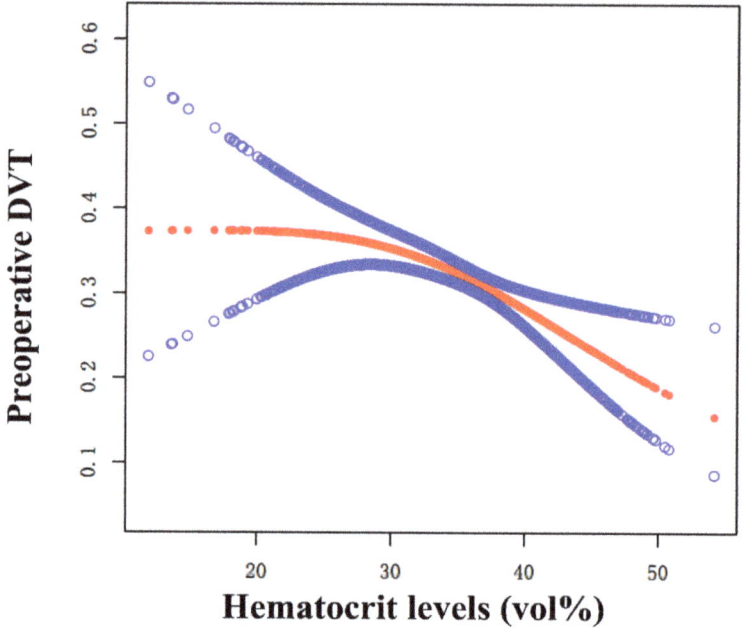

Figure 3. Curve fitting between admission hematocrit levels and preoperative DVT. Adjusted for sex, dementia, and multiple injuries.

Table 4. Nonlinearity of admission hematocrit levels versus preoperative DVT (N = 1840).

Outcome:	OR (95% CI) p-Value
Fitting model by standard linear regression	0.97 (0.95, 0.99) 0.0019
Fitting model by two-piecewise linear regression	
Inflection point	33.5 vol%
<33.5 vol%	1.00 (0.97, 1.04) 0.8230
>33.5 vol%	0.94 (0.91, 0.97) 0.0006
P for log-likelihood ratio test	0.029

Adjusted for sex, dementia, and multiple injuries.

4. Discussion

Our study shows that the level of hematocrit at admission is a strong predictor of preoperative DVT in older adults with hip fractures. Specifically, hematocrit levels at admission were nonlinearly associated with preoperative DVT. A hematocrit level of 33.5 vol% was the inflection point in the saturation effect. When the hematocrit level was <33.5 vol%, the hematocrit level at admission was not a potential risk factor for preoperative DVT (OR = 1.00), and the severity of low hematocrit was not associated with preoperative DVT. When the hematocrit level was >33.5 vol%, for each unit increase in hematocrit, the risk of preoperative DVT decreased by 6% (OR = 0.94). Therefore, a hematocrit level of 33.5 vol% is a useful indicator to predict preoperative DVT in older patients with hip fractures. In clinical practice, these findings can be used to identify high-risk patients who may benefit from specialized care.

Older adults with hip fractures are prone to DVT events due to advanced age, comorbidities (hypertension, heart disease, peripheral vascular disease, cerebrovascular disease), or risk factors (trauma, surgery, limb immobilization), further aggravating their poor prognosis. According to previous studies, the incidence of preoperative DVT in patients with hip fracture is 8–34.9%, and the incidence of DVT in patients with delayed surgery can even reach 62% [9,23,24]. A meta-analysis of 2022 analyzed 9823 patients and found that the incidence of preoperative DVT in elderly patients with hip fractures was 16.6%. Age, sex, BMI, low hemoglobin level, time from injury to admission, time from injury to surgery, type of hip fracture, CHD, dementia, pulmonary disease, kidney disease, smoking, fibrinogen, C-reactive protein, and albumin were considered independent risk factors for DVT [25].

Patients with polycythemia vera have been shown to be associated with an increased risk of DVT [26]. A Mendelian randomization study showed that a polygenic risk score for hemoglobin concentration was positively associated with venous thromboembolism risk in the general population [27]. Therefore, the hypothesis that detection of Hct levels has a predictive effect on the occurrence of DVT in elderly hip fractures has strong biological plausibility. The relationship between hematocrit levels and DVT incidence has previously been studied. A prospective study in Norway evaluating 26,108 adults showed that subjects with a hematocrit in the upper 20th percentile had a 1.5-fold higher risk of total DVT compared with subjects with a hematocrit in the lowest 40th percentile [19]. A case–control trial by Vayá et al. found that the proportion of subjects with a hematocrit greater than 45% was significantly higher in patients with DVT than in healthy controls [28]. A population-based cohort study from Denmark found a U-shaped association between Hct and VTE, but the association was not statistically significant [29]. A 2020 study showed that high levels of hematocrit and hemoglobin are associated with an increased long-term risk of VTE [18]. However, in a population-based longitudinal investigation of the etiology of thromboembolism, no significant association was reported between the hematocrit and the incidence of VTE [30]. An earlier case–control study also found no independent relationship between Hct and VTE [31]. Based on the above controversy, it remains to be further investigated whether hematocrit is the real cause of DVT or an innocent interloper, that is, whether the relationship between the two is causal or whether the relationship is confounded by other confounding factors [32].

Previous studies have been based on the general population. Results based on the general population are generally considered to have limited significance for specific populations. To our knowledge, this is the first study to investigate the relationship between hematocrit levels at admission and preoperative DVT in geriatric hip fractures. The prevalence of preoperative DVT in these patients is high (32%). We believe that previous studies may have underestimated the incidence of DVT. It is possible that the symptoms of hip fracture can mask the clinical signs and symptoms of DVT [33]. In this study, we established an association using curve fitting and found a saturation point and, therefore, a meaningful prediction point. Our study showed that hematocrit levels <33.5 vol% were not associated with preoperative DVT, whereas hematocrit levels at admission of >33.5 vol% were associated with preoperative DVT. Furthermore, according to the current anemia criteria, our study supports that anemia is a risk factor for developing DVT, and higher levels of HCT are associated with a lower risk of DVT.

To avoid the impact of COVID-19 on patient admission [34] and for a more accurate assessment of the relationship between hematocrit levels at admission and preoperative DVT, we performed linear regression on the adjusted model and comprehensively considered the variables that needed to be adjusted. Factors with $p < 0.1$ in the univariate analysis and factors included in previous studies were considered. Specifically, we used a sensitivity analysis of the trend test in the linear model. In addition, we considered the association of the curve and found a clinical saturation effect and an inflection point. Curve fitting was more suitable than linear fitting to explain the association between admission hematocrit levels and preoperative DVT.

Despite the large sample size and the many methods used to explain the relationship between variables and preoperative DVT, this study had several limitations. First, as with every other multivariate analysis, we were unable to include all confounding factors. Therefore, the residual confounding factors remained. Second, due to the limitations of the retrospective study design, we could not assess the progression of Hct levels over time. Third, our study was a single center study; all samples were from the same hospital, and hematocrit levels were strongly associated with region and ethnicity [35]. Therefore, these results should be interpreted with caution and the inference points for other ethnicities should be redefined.

In conclusion, hematocrit levels at admission were nonlinearly associated with preoperative DVT, and the hematocrit level at admission was a risk indicator of preoperative DVT. However, the severity of low hematocrit was not associated with preoperative DVT when the hematocrit was <33.5 vol%.

Author Contributions: According to the definition given by the International Committee of Medical Journal Editors (ICMJE), the authors listed above qualify for authorship based on making one or more substantial contributions to the intellectual content of the following: Conception and design of the study, B.-F.Z., Y.-M.Z., D.-Y.L., D.-X.L., T.Y. and K.-Y.Z.; analysis of the data, B.-F.Z. and D.-Y.L.; writing of the manuscript, D.-Y.L. All authors have read and agreed to the published version of the manuscript.

Funding: This work was supported by the Foundation of the Xi'an Municipal Health Commission (Grant Number: 2021ms09).

Institutional Review Board Statement: The study was conducted according to the Declaration of Helsinki guidelines and was approved by the Ethics Committee of Honghui Hospital, Xi'an Jiaotong University (protocol code: 202201009 and date of approval: 28 January 2022).

Informed Consent Statement: This study was registered on the website of the Chinese Clinical Trial Registry (ChiCTR: ChiCTR2200057323). Informed consent was obtained from all subjects involved in the study.

Data Availability Statement: Data were obtained from the Xi'an Honghui Hospital. According to relevant regulations, the data could not be shared but can be requested from the corresponding author.

Conflicts of Interest: The authors declare they have no conflict of interest.

Consent to Publish: The work described has not been published before (except in an abstract or as part of a published lecture, review, or thesis); it is not under consideration for publication elsewhere; and its publication has been approved by all co-authors.

Abbreviations

DVT	deep venous thrombosis
OR	odds ratio
CI	confidence interval
LMWH	low-molecular-weight heparin
CHD	coronary heart disease
COPD	chronic obstructive pulmonary disease
aCCI	age-adjusted Charlson comorbidity index

References

1. Gullberg, B.; Johnell, O.; Kanis, J. World-wide Projections for Hip Fracture. *Osteoporos. Int.* **1997**, *7*, 407–413. [CrossRef] [PubMed]
2. Veronese, N.; Maggi, S. Epidemiology and social costs of hip fracture. *Injury* **2018**, *49*, 1458–1460. [CrossRef] [PubMed]
3. Peeters, C.M.M.; Visser, E.; Van de Ree, C.L.P.; Gosens, T.; Den Oudsten, B.L.; De Vries, J. Quality of life after hip fracture in the elderly: A systematic literature review. *Injury* **2016**, *47*, 1369–1382. [CrossRef] [PubMed]
4. Koso, R.E.; Sheets, C.; Richardson, W.J.; Galanos, A.N. Hip Fracture in the Elderly Patients: A Sentinel Event. *Am. J. Hosp. Palliat. Med.* **2017**, *35*, 612–619. [CrossRef]
5. Meinberg, E.; Ward, D.; Herring, M.; Miclau, T. Hospital-based Hip fracture programs: Clinical need and effectiveness. *Injury* **2020**, *51*, S2–S4. [CrossRef]

6. Kaperonis, A.A.; Michelsen, C.B.; Askanazi, J.; Kinney, J.M.; Chien, S. Effects of Total Hip Replacement and Bed Rest on Blood Rheology and Red Cell Metabolism. *J. Trauma Inj. Infect. Crit. Care* **1988**, *28*, 453–457. [CrossRef]
7. Cho, Y.-H.; Byun, Y.-S.; Jeong, D.-G.; Han, I.-H.; Park, Y.-B. Preoperative Incidence of Deep Vein Thrombosis after Hip Fractures in Korean. *Clin. Orthop. Surg.* **2015**, *7*, 298–302. [CrossRef]
8. Luksameearunothai, K.; Sa-Ngasoongsong, P.; Kulachote, N.; Thamyongkit, S.; Fuangfa, P.; Chanplakorn, P.; Woratanarat, P.; Suphachatwong, C. Usefulness of clinical predictors for preoperative screening of deep vein thrombosis in hip fractures. *BMC Musculoskelet. Disord.* **2017**, *18*, 208. [CrossRef]
9. Shin, W.; Woo, S.; Lee, S.; Lee, J.; Kim, C.; Suh, K. Preoperative Prevalence of and Risk Factors for Venous Thromboembolism in Patients with a Hip Fracture: An Indirect Multidetector CT Venography Study. *J. Bone Jt. Surg. Am.* **2016**, *98*, 2089–2095. [CrossRef]
10. Song, K.; Yao, Y.; Rong, Z.; Shen, Y.; Zheng, M.; Jiang, Q. The preoperative incidence of deep vein thrombosis (DVT) and its correlation with postoperative DVT in patients undergoing elective surgery for femoral neck fractures. *Arch. Orthop. Trauma Surg.* **2016**, *136*, 1459–1464. [CrossRef]
11. Brill, J.B.; Badiee, J.; Zander, A.L.; Wallace, J.D.; Lewis, P.R.; Sise, M.J.; Bansal, V.; Shackford, S.R. The rate of deep vein thrombosis doubles in trauma patients with hypercoagulable thromboelastography. *J. Trauma Inj. Infect. Crit. Care* **2017**, *83*, 413–419. [CrossRef] [PubMed]
12. Ruskin, K. Deep vein thrombosis and venous thromboembolism in trauma. *Curr. Opin. Anaesthesiol.* **2018**, *31*, 215–218. [CrossRef] [PubMed]
13. Di Nisio, M.; van Es, N.; Buller, H. Deep vein thrombosis and pulmonary embolism. *Lancet* **2016**, *388*, 3060–3073. [CrossRef] [PubMed]
14. Long, A.; Zhang, L.; Zhang, Y.; Jiang, B.; Mao, Z.; Li, H.; Zhang, S.; Xie, Z.; Tang, P. Efficacy and safety of rivaroxaban versus low-molecular-weight heparin therapy in patients with lower limb fractures. *J. Thromb. Thrombolysis* **2014**, *38*, 299–305. [CrossRef] [PubMed]
15. Calder, J.D.F.; Freeman, R.; Domeij-Arverud, E.; Van Dijk, C.N.; Ackermann, P. Meta-analysis and suggested guidelines for prevention of venous thromboembolism (VTE) in foot and ankle surgery. *Knee Surg. Sport. Traumatol. Arthrosc.* **2016**, *24*, 1409–1420. [CrossRef] [PubMed]
16. Yavorkovsky, L.L. Mean corpuscular volume, hematocrit and polycythemia. *Hematology* **2021**, *26*, 881–884. [CrossRef]
17. Lowe, G.D.O.; Lee, A.J.; Rumley, A.; Price, J.F.; Fowkes, F.G.R. Blood viscosity and risk of cardiovascular events: The Edinburgh Artery Study. *Br. J. Haematol.* **1997**, *96*, 168–173. [CrossRef] [PubMed]
18. Folsom, A.; Wang, W.; Parikh, R.; Lutsey, P.; Beckman, J.; Cushman, M. Hematocrit and incidence of venous thromboembolism. *Res. Pract. Thromb. Haemost.* **2020**, *4*, 422–428. [CrossRef]
19. Braekkan, S.K.; Mathiesen, E.B.; Njølstad, I.; Wilsgaard, T.; Hansen, J.-B. Hematocrit and risk of venous thromboembolism in a general population. The Tromso study. *Haematologica* **2009**, *95*, 270–275. [CrossRef]
20. Zhang, B.; Wang, P.; Fei, C.; Shang, K.; Qu, S.; Li, J.; Ke, C.; Xu, X.; Yang, K.; Liu, P.; et al. Perioperative Deep Vein Thrombosis in Patients with Lower Extremity Fractures: An Observational Study, Clinical and applied thrombosis/hemostasis. *Off. J. Int. Acad. Clin. Appl. Thrombosis/Hemostasis* **2020**, *26*, 1076029620930272.
21. Mathew, G.; Agha, R.; Albrecht, J.; Goel, P.; Mukherjee, I.; Pai, P.; D'Cruz, A.K.; Nixon, I.J.; Roberto, K.; Enam, S.A.; et al. STROCSS 2021: Strengthening the reporting of cohort, cross-sectional and case-control studies in surgery. *Int. J. Surg.* **2021**, *96*, 106165. [CrossRef] [PubMed]
22. Mantoni, M. Ultrasound of limb veins. *Eur. Radiol.* **2001**, *11*, 1557–1562. [CrossRef] [PubMed]
23. Zhang, B.-F.; Wei, X.; Huang, H.; Wang, P.-F.; Liu, P.; Qu, S.-W.; Li, J.-H.; Wang, H.; Cong, Y.-X.; Zhuang, Y.; et al. Deep vein thrombosis in bilateral lower extremities after hip fracture: A retrospective study of 463 patients. *Clin. Interv. Aging* **2018**, *13*, 681–689. [CrossRef] [PubMed]
24. Smith, E.B.; Parvizi, J.; Purtill, J.J. Delayed Surgery for Patients with Femur and Hip Fractures—Risk of Deep Venous Thrombosis. *J. Trauma Inj. Infect. Crit. Care* **2011**, *70*, E113–E116. [CrossRef]
25. Wang, T.; Guo, J.; Long, Y.; Yin, Y.; Hou, Z. Risk factors for preoperative deep venous thrombosis in hip fracture patients: A meta-analysis, Journal of orthopaedics and traumatology. *Off. J. Ital. Soc. Orthop. Traumatol.* **2022**, *23*, 19. [CrossRef]
26. Griesshammer, M.; Kiladjian, J.-J.; Besses, C. Thromboembolic events in polycythemia vera. *Ann. Hematol.* **2019**, *98*, 1071–1082. [CrossRef]
27. Richardson, T.G.; Harrison, S.; Hemani, G.; Smith, G.D. An atlas of polygenic risk score associations to highlight putative causal relationships across the human phenome. *Elife* **2019**, *8*, e43657. [CrossRef]
28. Vayá, A.; Falcó, C.; Simó, M.; Ferrando, F.; Mira, Y.; Todolí, J.; España, F.; Corella, L. Influence of lipids and obesity on haemorheological parameters in patients with deep vein thrombosis. *Thromb. Haemost.* **2007**, *98*, 621–626.
29. Warny, M.; Helby, J.; Birgens, H.S.; Bojesen, S.E.; Nordestgaard, B.G. Arterial and venous thrombosis by high platelet count and high hematocrit: 108 521 individuals from the Copenhagen General Population Study. *J. Thromb. Haemost.* **2019**, *17*, 1898–1911. [CrossRef]
30. Tsai, A.; Cushman, M.; Rosamond, W.; Heckbert, S.; Polak, J.; Folsom, A. Cardiovascular risk factors and venous thromboembolism incidence: The longitudinal investigation of thromboembolism etiology. *Arch. Intern. Med.* **2002**, *162*, 1182–1189. [CrossRef]

31. Vayá, A.; Mira, Y.; Martínez, M.; Villa, P.; Ferrando, F.; Estellés, A.; Corella, L.; Aznar, J. Biological risk factors for deep vein thrombosis. *Clin. Hemorheol. Microcirc.* **2002**, *26*, 41–53. [PubMed]
32. Schreijer, A.J.; Reitsma, P.H.; Cannegieter, S.C. High hematocrit as a risk factor for venous thrombosis. Cause or innocent bystander? *Haematologica* **2010**, *95*, 182–184. [CrossRef] [PubMed]
33. Bengoa, F.; Vicencio, G.; Schweitzer, D.; Lira, M.; Zamora, T.; Klaber, I. High prevalence of deep vein thrombosis in elderly hip fracture patients with delayed hospital admission, European journal of trauma and emergency surgery. *Off. Publ. Eur. Trauma Soc.* **2020**, *46*, 913–917. [CrossRef] [PubMed]
34. Zhong, H.; Poeran, J.; Liu, J.; Wilson, L.A.; Memtsoudis, S.G. Hip fracture characteristics and outcomes during COVID-19: A large retrospective national database review. *Br. J. Anaesth.* **2021**, *127*, 15–22. [CrossRef] [PubMed]
35. Mondal, H.; Lotfollahzadeh, S. *Hematocrit, StatPearls*; StatPearls Publishing: Treasure Island, FL, USA, 2022.

Disclaimer/Publisher's Note: The statements, opinions and data contained in all publications are solely those of the individual author(s) and contributor(s) and not of MDPI and/or the editor(s). MDPI and/or the editor(s) disclaim responsibility for any injury to people or property resulting from any ideas, methods, instructions or products referred to in the content.

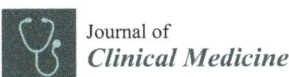

Article

What Are the Key Factors of Functional Outcomes in Patients with Spinopelvic Dissociation Treated with Triangular Osteosynthesis?

Po-Han Su [1,2], Yi-Hsun Huang [1,2], Chen-Wei Yeh [1,2], Chun-Yen Chen [2,3], Yuan-Shun Lo [2,4], Hsien-Te Chen [2] and Chun-Hao Tsai [1,2,5,*]

1. School of Medicine, China Medical University, Taichung 404, Taiwan
2. Department of Orthopedic Surgery, China Medical University Hospital, China Medical University, Taichung 404, Taiwan
3. Department of Orthopedic Surgery, Wei Gong Memorial Hospital, Miaoli 351, Taiwan
4. Department of Orthopedic Surgery, China Medical University Bei Gang Hospital, Yunlin 651, Taiwan
5. Department of Sports Medicine, College of Health Care, China Medical University, Taichung 404, Taiwan
* Correspondence: ritsai8615@gmail.com

Abstract: For patients with spinopelvic dissociation (SPD), triangular osteosynthesis is the current method for the fixation of the posterior pelvis. This study aimed to assess the recovery process and radiographic parameters associated with the functional outcomes in patients with SPD treated by triangular osteosynthesis. We collected data from 23 patients with SPD. To investigate the key aspect regarding the functional outcomes of these patients, we measured pre- and post-operative parameters, and a statistical analysis adjusted for age, gender, and time windows was used. The radiographic displacement measurement in the pre-operative period showed that the EQ−5D−5L increased by 2.141 per outlet ratio unit. The EQ−5D−5L increased by 1.359 per inlet ratio unit and 1.804 per outlet ratio during the postoperative period. The EQ−VAS increased significantly only with the inlet ratio in the postoperative period (1.270 per inlet ratio). A vertical reduction in SPD during the surgery can achieve more satisfactory outcomes than a horizontal anatomical reduction, in which the horizontal displacement causes inferior functional outcomes.

Keywords: spinopelvic dissociation; triangular osteosynthesis; functional outcome

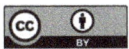

1. Introduction

Spinopelvic dissociation (SPD) is associated with transverse sacral fractures, which cause the dissociation of the sacrum from the pelvis [1,2]. It is associated with 3% of transverse sacral fractures and 3% of sacral fractures are associated with pelvic ring injuries [3]. SPD is well known for its high mortality and comorbidities such as nerve root injuries [4]. When SPD is correctly diagnosed and appropriately treated, patient outcomes can be optimized [5]. However, a high level of consensus and a unified approach for dealing with this complex issue are lacking.

The traditional fixation methods for the posterior pelvic ring include tension band transiliac plate fixation, local plate fixation, open or percutaneous ilio-sacral screw fixation, and transiliac bars, which do not guarantee postoperative stability and may result in fixation failures [6,7]. In recent years, surgeons have used triangular osteosynthesis (TOS) in combination with the surgical technique of unilateral L5 fixation using S2AI or iliac screws for SPD treatment, and the literature indicates that these patients show satisfactory postoperative function and radiological outcomes [8]. With or without a combination of bilateral or dual iliac screw fixation techniques [9], TOS is a reliable form of fixation that enables early weight-bearing while preventing the loss of reduction [9–12]. In addition, compared with traditional surgical methods, its complication rate is low [3,5] (Figure 1A–F).

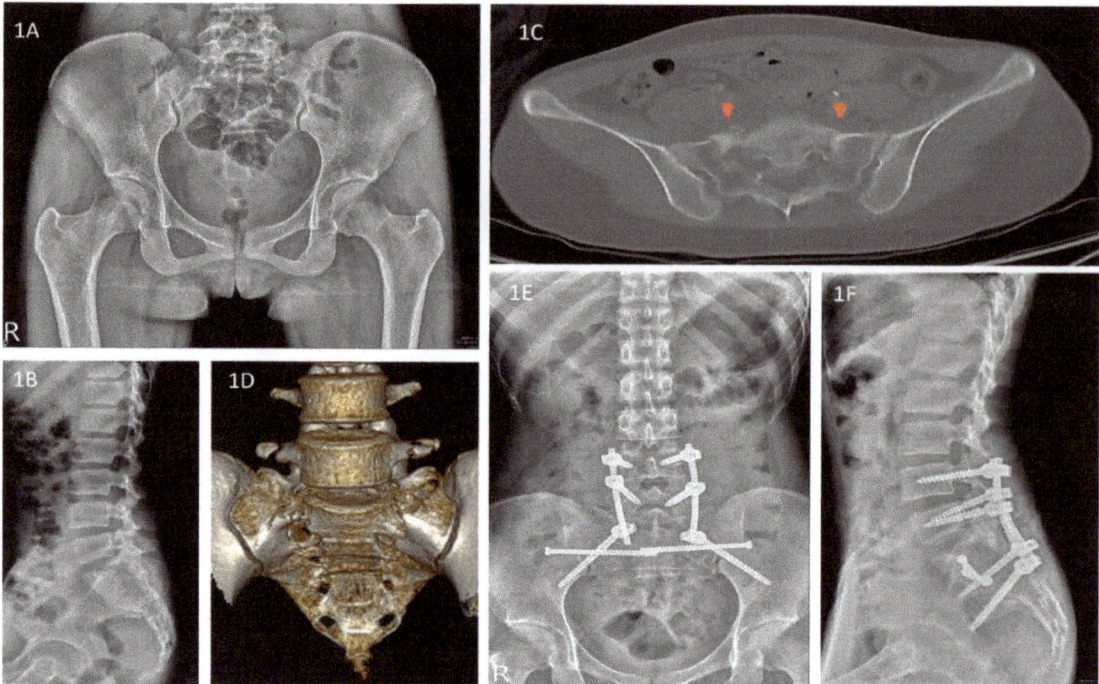

Figure 1. (**A–F**) Pre- and postoperative radiography and CT images of a 21-year-old woman who fell from a bridge and developed bifrontal EDH, facial bone fractures, and bilateral sacral fractures with spinopelvic dissociation that were presented in the emergency room. (**A**) AP view of the pelvis on admission showing bilateral fracture lines on the sacrum; (**B**) lateral view of the sacral spine view on admission showing fracture lines on the sacrum, indicating displaced fragments over the fracture site; (**C**) axial CT view of the sacrum demonstrating bilateral fracture lines indicating U-type sacral fractures; (**D**) 3D CT view of the sacrum demonstrating a displaced U-shape sacral fracture (red arrows) and AO/OTA 54C3 type, Denis Zone II sacral fracture; (**E**) Postoperative AP pelvic view: the sacral fracture was stabilized by bilateral triangular osteosynthesis with S2AI screws. (**F**) Postoperative lateral view of the sacral spine: The trajectory of S2AI screws was set under O-arm navigation to obtain an optimal length. Abbreviations: EDH = epidural hematoma, CT = computed tomography, and AP = anteroposterior.

Currently, a radiographic assessment remains the standard peri-operative measurement for displacement and reduction in studies of pelvic fractures. However, there is still a lack of research investigating the relationship between peri-operative SPD and prognosis from the perspective of radiology in patients with SPD who underwent reduction and fixation by TOS using S2AI screws. Though the measurement of outcomes is difficult and the level of evidence in this area is poor, this article revealed three such methods for measuring radiographic displacement [11,13,14].

This study aimed to investigate the recovery time course and imaging parameters relevant to the functional recovery of patients with SPD treated by TOS.

2. Materials and Methods

2.1. Patient Selection and Classification

This is an observational, retrospective study. From August 2018 to September 2021, 29 patients with SPD were recruited. One was excluded due to severe spinal cord injuries, and five were lost to follow-up in our orthopedic clinic department. Complete series of pre-and post-operative radiographs were collected from the remaining 23 patients who suffered pelvic fractures with SPD treated by TOS fixation using the S2AI screw fixation technique. To make the procedure more appropriate and to obtain an optimal length and deflection angle, we set the trajectory of the S2AI screws under O-arm navigation (Figure 2A–F) [15]. These patients were postoperatively followed-up for a minimum of one year in the clinic as a single cohort. The study protocol was approved by the Research Ethics Committee of the China Medical University Hospital, Taichung, Taiwan (protocol ID: CMUH108−REC3−144) and conducted in accordance with the ethical principles of the Helsinki Declaration. The inclusion criteria include skeletally mature patients who suffered pelvic fractures with SPD treated by TOS fixation. Based on the anatomic relationship between the fracture site and the sacral neural foramen, Denis et al. classified sacral fractures into three types. Roy-Camille et al. classified transverse sacral fractures of the Denis III zone into three subtypes based on the degree of displacement and the traumatic mechanism [16,17]. In this study, most patients were in Denis zones I and II.

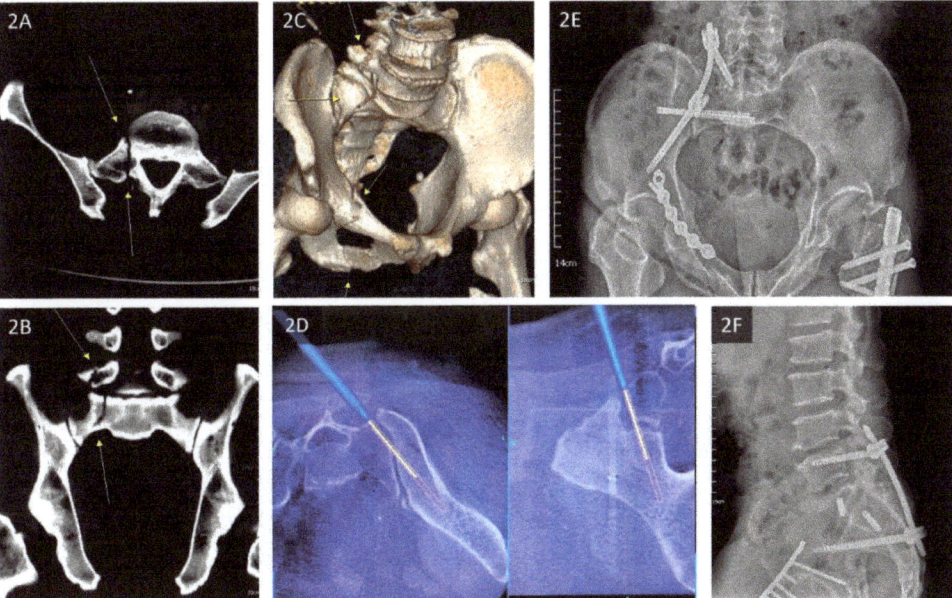

Figure 2. (**A**–**F**) Pre- and postoperative radiography and CT images of a 56-year-old man who was hit by a vehicle and had right superior and inferior rami fractures, a right L5 transverse process fracture, and a right sacral fracture with spinopelvic dissociation. The associated injury included a left femoral shaft fracture, right femoral shaft segmental fracture, and left medial malleolar fracture. (**A**) Axial CT view of the sacrum on admission demonstrating fracture lines (yellow arrows) over the right L5 transverse process; (**B**) coronal CT view of the sacrum on admission demonstrating fracture lines (yellow arrows) over the right sacrum; (**C**) 3D CT view of the pelvis showing right superior and inferior rami fractures (yellow arrows), a right L5 transverse process fracture (yellow arrows), and a right AO/OTA 61C1.3 and 54B3 type, Denis Zone II, sacral fracture (yellow arrows); (**D**) with the assistance of O-arm navigation, the optimal trajectory of the S2AI screw was set (O-arm and Stealth Station S7 Surgical Navigation System, Stryker); (**E**) postoperative view of the inlet pelvis—the sacral fracture was stabilized by triangular osteosynthesis with S2AI screws, and the right superior rami fracture was reduced and fixed with a pre-contoured locking plate; (**F**) postoperative lateral view of the sacral spine. Abbreviations: CT = computed tomography.

2.2. Radiographic Methods

To assess the imaging parameters associated with the functional recovery, we used three radiographic methods and three functional outcome questionnaires in this study.

Three experienced orthopedic trauma surgeons collaborated on this measurement plan and independently measured radiographic features. For measurements using computer-based-reading methods, each observer was given an identical set of images (pre- and postoperative anteroposterior (AP), outlet, and inlet views). This study aimed to investigate the correlation between radiological measurements and the functional outcome. Three previously published radiographic measurement methods were chosen. Each observer was provided with a set of images (23 patients and six images per patient) and received the same instructions for measurement, including three radiographic measurement methods, which are described below (Table 1).

Table 1. Radiographic measurement methods for assessment of displacement and symmetry for pelvic fracture with spinopelvic dissociation.

Authors	Methods	Description
Sagi et al., 2009	Inlet and outlet ratio Method (Sagi Method) [11]	On the inlet view, we drew a line across the anterior border of the sacrum, perpendicular to the spinous processes. The perpendicular distance from this line to the subchondral bone of each acetabulum was measured, and a ratio was then calculated, with the affected side of pelvis set as the numerator. A similar ratio was obtained for the outlet view by drawing a line parallel to the superior end plate of S1, perpendicular to the spinous processes. The perpendicular distance from the reference line to the subchondral bone of each acetabulum was measured, and a ratio was then calculated, with the affected side of pelvis set as the numerator (Figure 3).
Keshishyan et al., 1995	Cross measurement method (Keshishyan Method) [14]	The measurement method described by Keshishyan et al. for assessing the displacement of pelvic ring continuity in children used only the AP pelvic view. Originally, this method was applied for skeletally immature patients and measures the distance from the inferior aspect of the sacroiliac (SI) joint to the contralateral triradiate cartilage. We used the modified method described by Lefaivre et al. to assess our adult patients. Observers were instructed to measure from the inferior SI joint (iliac side) to the inferior aspect of the teardrop in the AP pelvic view. "Y" was the length from the left SI joint to the right teardrop, and "X" was the opposite. Observers were instructed to measure the distance using the measuring software. We then calculated the ratio (X/Y) to standardize the baseline of comparison of the displacement (Figure 4).
Lefaivre et al., 2009	Absolute displacement method (ADM) [13]	This method was initially proposed by Lefaivre et al. in 2009. Observers were instructed to use preoperative pelvic AP, inlet, and outlet views. In each view, a horizontal line was drawn across the superior end plate of L5 as a reference line. If this was not visible in the film, the observers were asked to use the inferior end plate of L5 as a reference. Measurements were either parallel or perpendicular to this reference line. This line was used as the direction for horizontal measurements, or a line 90 degrees to this reference line was used for vertical measurements. Maximum displacements in the anterior and posterior pelvic rings were measured in each plane film. After completing the six measurements of the three preoperative films (anterior and posterior rings in each of the AP, outlet, and inlet views), the observers were instructed to measure the same anatomic locations in the postoperative plane films. Finally, the largest single measurements from the six preoperative and postoperative measurements were considered the preoperative and postoperative maximum displacements, respectively (Figure 5A,B).

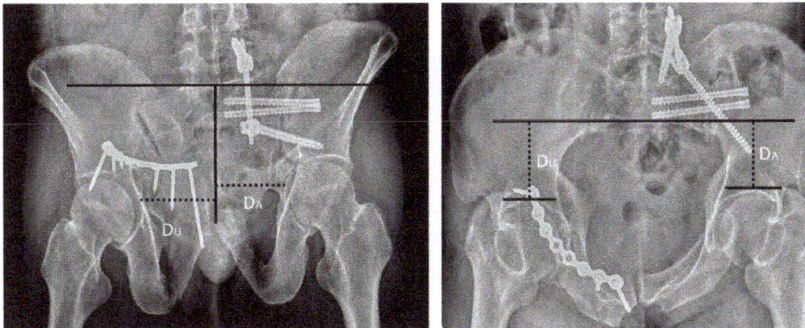

Figure 3. The inlet and outlet ratio are calculated (DA/DU) with the pelvic inlet and outlet views. The solid lines refer the reference lines, and the dashed lines refer measured lines. The Abbreviations: DA = distance of affected side; DU = distance of unaffected side.

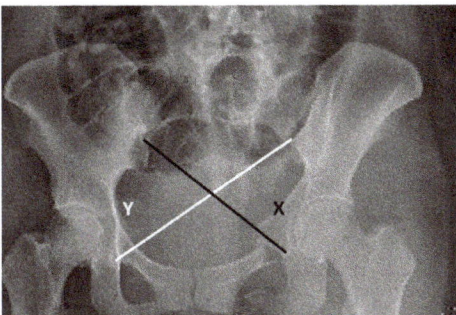

Figure 4. The cross—measurement method is illustrated with an example image.

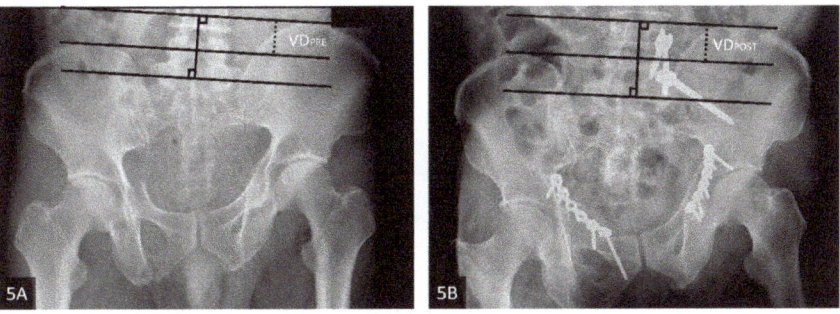

Figure 5. (**A,B**) The absolute displacement method (ADM). The example image illustrated the measurement of vertical displacement in pelvis AP view pre- and post-operatively. (**A**) Pre-operative pelvis AP view. (**B**) Post-operative pelvis AP view. The reference lines are solid, and the measured lines are dashed. The Abbreviations: VDPRE = the pre-operative vertical displacement; VDPOST = the post-operative vertical displacement.

2.3. Statistical Methods

Numbers (percentages) were used to represent the distribution of gender, AO 2018 classification, and Denis zone [16]. The mean (standard deviation [SD]) and median (interquartile range [IQR]) were used to show the distribution of age, the radiographic displacement measurement (including the inlet ratio, outlet ratio, deformity index, asymmetry, deformity ratio, vertical displacement [VD], and horizontal displacement [HD]) in pre- and postoperative periods, VD change (preoperative minus postoperative values), and HD change (preoperative minus postoperative values). Generalized estimating equations (GEE) were used to estimate differences in outcomes (including the EQ−5D−5L [18], EQ−VAS, and Majeed pelvic scores [19]) among different time windows. The model was adjusted for age and gender. We also used the GEE model to assess the association between outcomes and different radiographic displacement measurements. The model was adjusted for age, gender, and time windows.

3. Results

As shown in Table 2, a total of 23 patients were enrolled in this study. There were 15 men and 8 women (65.2% vs. 34.8%), and the mean age was 47.8 (19.3) years. More than half of the patients were in the 61C1 (60.9%) category according to the AO 2018 classification, followed by those in the 61C3 (26.1%), 61C2 (8.70%), and 62C2 (4.35%) categories.

Table 2. Patients' characteristics (*n* = 12).

Variable	n (%)	
Men	15 (65.2%)	
Women	8 (34.8%)	
AO 2018 classification		
61C1	14 (60.9%)	
61C2	2 (8.70%)	
61C3	6 (26.1%)	
62C2	1 (4.35%)	
Denis zone		
I	10 (43.5%)	
II	10 (43.5%)	
III	3 (13.0%)	
	Mean (SD)	Median (IQR)
Age (years)	47.8 (19.3)	47.0 (32.0)
Preoperative		
Inlet ratio	0.90 (0.07)	0.91 (0.11)
Outlet ratio	0.96 (0.10)	0.85 (0.10)
Deformity index	0.04 (0.04)	0.04 (0.05)
Asymmetry	12.6 (11.0)	10.6 (13.1)
Deformity ratio	0.94 (0.10)	0.94 (0.10)
VD	14.9 (14.7)	12.6 (13.3)
HD	13.0 (13.7)	6.65 (18.3)
Postoperative		
Inlet ratio	0.92 (0.07)	0.92 (0.06)
Outlet ratio	0.91 (0.08)	0.92 (0.11)
Deformity index	0.05 (0.06)	0.04 (0.05)
Asymmetry	11.9 (9.71)	10.1 (15.0)
Deformity ratio	0.91 (0.10)	0.93 (0.10)
VD	6.99 (11.1)	4.33 (9.90)
HD	7.33 (8.75)	3.81 (13.4)
VD change	7.46 (5.22)	7.73 (7.12)
HD change	7.63 (5.25)	7.95 (7.33)

Abbreviations: SD = standard deviation, IQR = interquartile range, VD = vertical displacement, and HD = horizontal displacement.

As time progressed, the functional outcomes improved, and the patients returned to a near-normal life within one year. The EQ−5D−5L score increased with time, from 0.14 at 6–8 weeks to 0.94 at one year. The differences for the time trend were 0.32 in the crude GEE model (95% confidence interval [CI]: 0.25, 0.39) and 0.31 in the adjusted GEE model (95% CI: 0.25, 0.37) (Table 3, Figure 6). The EQ−VAS and Majeed pelvic scores also increased with time. The differences for the time trend were 0.17 for the EQ−VAS (95% CI: 0.14, 0.30) and 0.20 for the Majeed pelvic score in the adjusted GEE model (95% CI: 0.18, 0.22).

Table 3. Distribution of outcomes among time windows.

	EQ−5D−5L	EQ−VAS	Majeed Pelvic Score
Variable	Mean (SD)	Mean (SD)	Mean (SD)
Time window			
6–8 weeks	0.14 (0.43)	51.2 (11.7)	49.2 (9.32)
3 months	0.46 (0.28)	63.7 (15.9)	60.1 (13.2)
6 months	0.74 (0.16)	77.5 (15.9)	77.5 (15.2)
1 year	0.94 (0.09)	92.3 (9.32)	94.5 (8.12)
Crude estimated (95% CI)	0.32 (0.25, 0.39)	0.17 (0.14, 0.20)	0.20 (0.18, 0.22)
p-value	<0.0001	<0.0001	<0.0001
* Adjusted estimated (95% CI)	0.31 (0.25, 0.37)	0.17 (0.14, 0.20)	0.20 (0.18, 0.22)
* p-value	<0.0001	<0.0001	<0.0001

* Adjusted for age and gender in the GEE model. Abbreviations: SD = standard deviation, CI = confidence interval, and GEE = Generalized estimating equations.

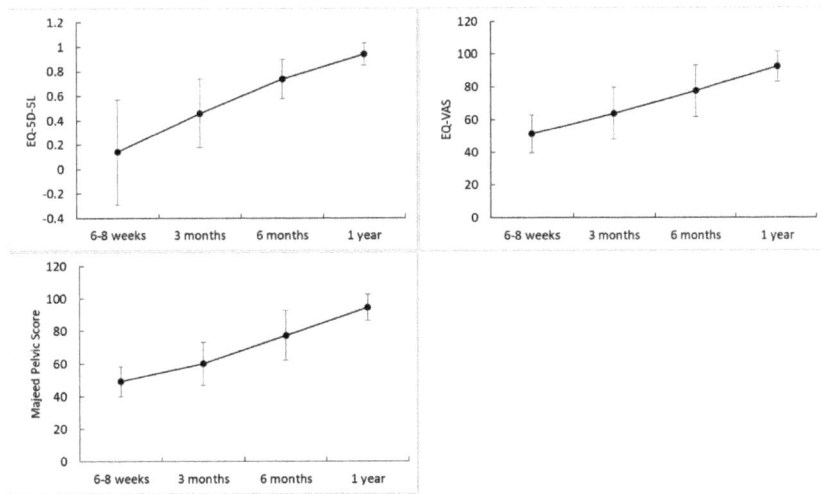

Figure 6. EQ−5D−5L, EQ−VAS, and Majeed pelvic scores over time.

In this study, three image-evaluation methods, including the measurement of the inlet–outlet ratio, the cross−measurement method, and ADM, were used pre-and postoperatively. The association between the EQ−5D−5L score and the radiographic displacement measurement is presented in Table 4. For the preoperative radiographic displacement measurements, the EQ−5D−5L score increased by 2.141 per outlet ratio unit (95% CI: 0.041, 4.241). In the postoperative period, the EQ−5D−5L score increased by 1.359 per inlet ratio unit and 1.804 per outlet ratio (95% CI: 1.301, 2.307) but decreased by 0.01 per HD (95% CI: −0.018, −0.002) after adjusting for age, gender, and the follow-up time. This shows that changes in the horizontal direction are more correlated with EQ−5D−5L recovery.

Table 4. Association between EQ−5D−5L scores and measurements in the GEE model.

Variable	Crude Estimated (95% CI)	p-Value	* Adjusted Estimated (95% CI)	** p-Value
Preoperative				
Inlet ratio	0.948 (−1.492, 3.388)	0.446	1.013 (−0.275, 2.300)	0.123
Outlet ratio	2.409 (0.838, 3.981)	0.003	2.141 (0.041, 4.241)	0.046 **
Deformity index	1.530 (−0.359, 3.419)	0.112	0.614 (−1.428, 2.656)	0.556
Asymmetry	0.005 (−0.005, 0.014)	0.327	0.002 (−0.007, 0.010)	0.728
Deformity ratio	0.344 (−0.936, 1.623)	0.599	−0.314 (−1.121, 0.493)	0.446
VD	0.002 (−0.002, 0.007)	0.371	−0.002 (−0.006, 0.003)	0.461
HD	−0.001 (−0.009, 0.008)	0.845	−0.002 (−0.010, 0.007)	0.673
Postoperative				
Inlet ratio	1.157 (−1.204, 3.519)	0.337	1.359 (0.144, 2.574)	0.028 **
Outlet ratio	1.605 (0.184 3.026)	0.027	1.804 (1.301, 2.307)	<0.0001 **
Deformity index	0.755 (−0.219, 1.728)	0.129	−0.994 (−2.093, 0.106)	0.077
Asymmetry	−0.007 (−0.019, 0.006)	0.321	−0.008 (−0.019, 0.003)	0.144
Deformity ratio	−0.350 (−1.105, 0.405)	0.363	0.651 (−0.005, 1.301)	0.052
VD	0.003 (−0.003, 0.009)	0.365	−0.004 (−0.010, 0.002)	0.215
HD	−0.009 (−0.020, 0.002)	0.105	−0.010 (−0.018, −0.002)	0.010 **
VD change	0.009 (−0.011, 0.029)	0.388	0.008 (−0.008, 0.023)	0.331
HD change	0.006 (−0.014, 0.027)	0.544	0.007 (−0.009, 0.022)	0.402

* Adjusted for age, sex, and time window. ** p-values < 0.05 represent statistical significance. Abbreviations: GEE = Generalized estimating equations, CI = confidence interval, VD = vertical displacement, and HD = horizontal displacement.

The association between the EQ−VAS score and the radiographic displacement measurements is shown in Table 5. The association was significant only with the inlet ratio in the postoperative period. The EQ−VAS score increased by 1.270 per inlet ratio (95% CI: 0.093, 2.447) in the adjusted GEE model. However, there were no significant associations between the Majeed pelvic score and any of the radiographic displacement measurements (Table 6).

Table 5. Associations between the EQ−VAS score and measurements in the GEE model.

Variable	Crude Estimated (95% CI)	p-Value	* Adjusted Estimated (95% CI)	** p-Value
Preoperative				
Inlet ratio	0.733 (−1.173, 2.640)	0.451	0.463 (−0.393, 1.318)	0.289.
Outlet ratio	1.299 (0.591, 2.008)	0.0003	0.330 (−0.240, 0.900)	0.256
Deformity index	1.122 (−0.830, 3.073)	0.260	0.623 (−1.076, 2.322)	0.472
Asymmetry	0.002 (−0.009, 0.013)	0.700	0.001 (−0.008, 0.009)	0.822
Deformity ratio	0.464 (−0.881, 1.810)	0.499	−0.308 (−0.957, 0.341)	0.353
VD	0.003 (−0.004, 0.009)	0.453	−0.0007 (−0.004, 0.03)	0.693
HD	−0.002 (−0.008, 0.005)	0.593	−0.002 (−0.007, 0.003)	0.377
Postoperative				
Inlet ratio	1.233 (−0.879, 3.345)	0.252	1.270 (0.093, 2.447)	0.034 **
Outlet ratio	0.551 (−0.047, 1.549)	0.279	0.455 (−0.365, 1.274)	0.277
Deformity index	1.027 (0.017, 2.037)	0.046	−0.383 (−1.042, 0.276)	0.255
Asymmetry	−0.004 (−0.014, 0.006)	0.432	−0.003 (−0.009, 0.004)	0.459
Deformity ratio	−0.460 (−1.316, 0.396)	0.292	0.203 (−0.184, 0.590)	0.303
VD	0.005 (−0.002, 0.011)	0.197	−0.0002 (−0.004, 0.003)	0.927
HD	−0.003 (−0.009, 0.004)	0.436	−0.004 (−0.010, 0.001)	0.130
VD change	−0.003 (−0.026, 0.019)	0.779	−0.005 (−0.022, 0.012)	0.572
HD change	−0.005 (−0.027, 0.018)	0.688	−0.005 (−0.023, 0.012)	0.555

* Adjusted for age, sex, and time window; ** p-values < 0.05, representing statistical significance. Abbreviations: GEE = Generalized estimating equations, CI = confidence interval, VD = vertical displacement, and HD = horizontal displacement.

Table 6. Association between the Majeed Pelvic Score and measurements in the GEE model.

Variable	Crude Estimated (95% CI)	p-Value	* Adjusted Estimated (95% CI)	** p-Value
Preoperative				
Inlet ratio	0.937 (−0.463, 2.337)	0.190	0.714 (−0.134, 1.562)	0.099
outlet ratio	0.790 (0.038, 1.542)	0.040	0.009 (−0.579, 0.600)	0.977
Deformity index	0.618 (−1.354, 2.589)	0.539	0.030 (−1.932, 1.991)	0.976
Asymmetry	0.0004 (−0.010, 0.011)	0.942	−0.001 (−0.010, 0.008)	0.763
Deformity ratio	0.168 (−0.772, 1.108)	0.726	−0.207 (−0.811, 0.396)	0.501
VD	0.0004 (−0.004, 0.004)	0.856	−0.001 (−0004, 0.003)	0.586
HD	−0.001 (−0.008, 0.006)	0.868	−0.001 (−0.007, 0.005)	0.716
Postoperative				
Inlet ratio	1.126 (−0.414, 2.665)	0.152	0.871 (−0.376, 2.117)	0.171
outlet ratio	0.528 (−0.238, 1.294)	0.177	0.342 (−0.422, 1.105)	0.381
Deformity index	0.186 (−0.628, 1.000)	0.654	−0.641 (−1.415, 0.133)	0.105
Asymmetry	−0.005 (−0.013, 0.003)	0.201	−0.003 (−0.010, 0.003)	0.322
Deformity ratio	−0.038 (−0.612, 0.535)	0.896	0.365 (−0.090, 0.820)	0.115
VD	0.001 (−0.003, 0.005)	0.582	−0.001 (−0.005, 0.002)	0.441
HD	−0.004 (−0.010, 0.002)	0.171	−0.004 (−0.010, 0.002)	0.199
VD change	−0.002 (−0.025, 0.021)	0876	−0.003 (−0.023, 0.017)	0.794
HD change	−0.003 (−0.026, 0.020)	0.814	−0.003 (−0.023, 0.018)	0.798

* Adjusted for age, sex, and time window; ** p-values < 0.05, representing statistical significance. Abbreviations: GEE = Generalized estimating equations, CI = confidence interval, VD = vertical displacement, and HD = horizontal displacement.

4. Discussion

The present study revealed that the displacement of SPD in spinopelvic fixation provides good vertical reduction results. During surgery, a reduction in the vertical direction is easier to achieve by fluoroscopy. A vertical anatomical reduction is often mentioned and highlighted for the treatment of unequal feet. A vertical displacement causes differences in the lower extremities, abnormal motor gaits, and lower Majeed scores.

It is sometimes difficult to achieve a perfect horizontal reduction due to comminuted sacroiliac fractures or an indirect reduction in the sacroiliac joints with complex anatomical structures radiologically.

Regarding horizontal reduction, the analysis showed that patients with a short-term follow-up showed a lower tolerance for postoperative horizontal displacement. Only a few studies have focused on the relationship between the inferior quality of horizontal displacement reduction and unsatisfying functional outcomes. We believe that the inferior quality of the horizontal reduction results in a change in the lever arm of the peak moment of the hip, which causes greater work in terms of hip abduction, adduction, flexion, and extension in the affected side in patients with SPD (Figure 7). As a result, the centroid experiences a mid-lateral shift, which may increase the metabolic cost and mechanical work of the lower extremities [20,21]. With rehabilitation, patients improved their function over time, but the change of the lever arm may contribute to unsatisfaction, increasing metabolic costs, and increased mechanical work in the short term postoperatively. No significant correlation was found in the asymmetric index. This could be because the integrity of the pelvic ring was restored postoperatively, while the SI joint was left without a complete reduction.

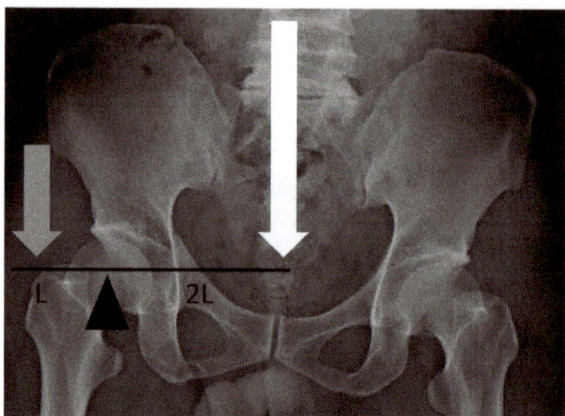

Figure 7. Coronal view of the hip illustrating the change of the lever arm around the hip's center. When we set the hip's center as a fulcrum, there are two opposing forces across the hip's center: the body weight (white arrow) and abductor muscles (gray arrow). The lever arm for body weight is longer. In patients with SPD, horizontal displacement of the hip's center often extends the lever arm for body weight, causing increased work to balance the moment.

Our results revealed that the patient's function will return to normal in one year. The postoperative gait analyses of patients with various pelvic ring fractures by Kubota et al. [22,23] showed that there was a complete recovery of peak hip abduction, and a partial recovery of peak hip extension and hip strength were noted at the 12-month follow-up. The horizontal displacement of the pelvis may affect the offset change of the hip joint, which is associated with abductor function. Dean et al. [24] concluded that patients with type C pelvic fractures had weaker hip abductor strengths, lower peak hip abduction moments, slower walking speeds, lower peak hip abductions, and lower peak hip extensions in the short-term after the surgery; however, at the 12-month follow-up, the bilateral hip strength (abduction, adduction, flexion, and extension), bilateral peak hip moment (abduction, adduction, flexion, and extension), peak hip power, or walking speed did not differ between groups. We reasoned that an insufficient hip abduction strength may in turn lead to differences in short-term functional outcomes [22–24].

There is no perfect assessment tool, and the measurements of pelvic radiographs have not yet been well validated [25]. This is the first study to connect functional outcomes to radiological assessments. We found that the questionnaires and assessment tools for functional outcomes were often subjective and generalized; therefore, currently, we can hardly ascribe the unsatisfying hip function to the postoperative horizontal residual displacement. Although reduction is important, the evaluation of the association between the radiological displacement and functional outcomes requires better tools. In patients with SPD, there will be multi-axial displacements, including horizontal, vertical, and rotational displacements. The plain radiographs could only reveal the measurement of horizontal or vertical displacements, whereas the rotational displacement could be assessed by CT. It is reported that CT or three-dimensional reconstruction-based displacement measurements of pelvic ring injury displacement may provide a more accurate assessment [26].

This study had some limitations. First, a tomographic analysis is warranted to assess the rotation, but a customized view along the long axis of the pelvic bone is required for a correct assessment. Second, this was a single-center, observational, retrospective study with a small number of participants. However, as patients suffering from pelvic fractures with SPD are relatively rare, greater-scale research is difficult to carry out. To improve patients' functional outcomes and satisfaction, this study sets a template for future research focusing on this topic. Further studies with more patient data would help to improve the understanding of the correlation between the functional outcomes and reductions in different dimensions.

5. Conclusions

TOS is a powerful fixation technique for patients with SPD. We achieved the vertical reduction in SPD more easily through fluoroscopy during the operation than with horizontal anatomical reduction, while horizontal displacement caused inferior satisfaction.

Author Contributions: Conceptualization, P.-H.S. and C.-H.T.; methodology, P.-H.S. and C.-H.T.; validation, P.-H.S. and C.-H.T.; formal analysis, C.-H.T.; investigation, P.-H.S., Y.-H.H. and C.-W.Y.; resources, C.-Y.C., Y.-S.L., H.-T.C. and C.-H.T.; data curation, P.-H.S.; writing—original draft preparation, P.-H.S.; writing—review and editing, C.-H.T.; visualization, C.-H.T.; supervision, H.-T.C. and C.-H.T.; project administration, C.-H.T. All authors have read and agreed to the published version of the manuscript.

Funding: This research received no external funding.

Institutional Review Board Statement: The observational retrospective study protocol was approved by the Research Ethics Committee of the China Medical University Hospital, Taichung, Taiwan (protocol ID: CMUH108-REC3-144).

Informed Consent Statement: Informed consent was obtained from all subjects involved in the study.

Data Availability Statement: Not applicable.

Acknowledgments: The authors would like to thank all colleagues who contributed to this study. We are grateful to Hsiang-Wen Lin, for her collaboration and providing the Traditional Chinese (Taiwan) Version of the EQ-5D-5L Questionnaire during preliminary investigations, and to Chiu Yu Shih, in the orthopedics department of Changhua Christian hospital, who assisted with the IRB approval of this study.

Conflicts of Interest: The authors declare no conflict of interest.

References

1. Yi, C.; Hak, D.J. Traumatic spinopelvic dissociation or U-shaped sacral fracture: A review of the literature. *Injury* **2012**, *43*, 402–408. [CrossRef]
2. Strange-Vognsen, H.H.; Lebech, A. An unusual type of fracture in the upper sacrum. *J. Orthop. Trauma* **1991**, *5*, 200–203. [CrossRef] [PubMed]
3. Quacinella, M.A.; Morrissey, P.B.; Parry, J.A.; Mauffrey, C. Spinopelvic Dissociation: Assessment, Reduction Strategies, and Fixation Techniques. *J. Am. Acad. Orthop. Surg.* **2020**, *28*, e1086–e1096. [CrossRef]
4. Petryla, G.; Bobina, R.; Uvarovas, V.; Kurtinaitis, J.; Sveikata, T.; Ryliškis, S.; Kvederas, G.; Šatkauskas, I. Functional outcomes and quality of life after surgical treatment of spinopelvic dissociation: A case series with one-year follow-up. *BMC Musculoskelet. Disord.* **2021**, *22*, 795. [CrossRef] [PubMed]
5. Erkan, S.; Cetinarslan, O.; Okcu, G. Traumatic spinopelvic dissociation managed with bilateral triangular osteosynthesis: Functional and radiological outcomes, health related quality of life and complication rates. *Injury* **2021**, *52*, 95–101. [CrossRef] [PubMed]
6. Sakti, Y.M.; Mafaza, A.; Lanodiyu, Z.A.; Sakadewa, G.P.; Magetsari, R. Management of complex pelvic fracture and sacral fracture Denis type 2 using spanning unilateral fixation of L5 to S2AI screw. *Int. J. Surg. Case Rep.* **2020**, *77*, 543–548. [CrossRef]
7. Tisano, B.K.; Kelly, D.P.; Starr, A.J.; Sathy, A.K. Vertical shear pelvic ring injuries: Do transsacral screws prevent fixation failure? *OTA Int.* **2020**, *3*, e084. [CrossRef]
8. Berber, O.; Amis, A.A.; Day, A.C. Biomechanical testing of a concept of posterior pelvic reconstruction in rotationally and vertically unstable fractures. *J. Bone Jt. Surg.* **2011**, *93*, 237–244. [CrossRef]
9. Wanner, J.P.; Tatman, L.; Stephens, B.; Mitchell, P. Team Approach: Spinopelvic Dissociation. *JBJS Rev.* **2021**, *9*, e20. [CrossRef]
10. Santolini, E.; Kanakaris, N.K.; Giannoudis, P.V. Sacral fractures: Issues, challenges, solutions. *EFORT Open Rev.* **2020**, *5*, 299–311. [CrossRef]
11. Sagi, H.C.; Militano, U.; Caron, T.; Lindvall, E. A Comprehensive Analysis With Minimum 1-Year Follow-up of Vertically Unstable Transforaminal Sacral Fractures Treated With Triangular Osteosynthesis. *J. Orthop. Trauma* **2009**, *23*, 313–319. [CrossRef] [PubMed]
12. Tian, D.; Guo, X.; Liu, N.; Wang, B.; He, H.; Xiong, M. A Modified Triangular Osteosynthesis Protocol for the Rod and Pedicle Screw Fixation of Vertical Unstable Sacral Fractures. *Int. J. Spine Surg.* **2021**, *15*, 485–493. [CrossRef]
13. Lefaivre, K.A.; Starr, A.J.; Barker, B.; Overturf, S.; Reinert, C.M. Early experience with reduction of displaced disruption of the pelvic ring using a pelvic reduction frame. *J. Bone Jt. Surg.* **2009**, *91*, 1201–1207. [CrossRef] [PubMed]

14. Keshishyan, R.A.; Rozinov, V.M.; Malakhov, O.A.; Kuznetsov, L.E.; Strunin, E.G.; Chogovadze, G.A.; Tsukanov, V.E. Pelvic polyfractures in children. Radiographic diagnosis and treatment. *Clin. Orthop. Relat. Res.* **1995**, *320*, 28–33.
15. Zhao, Y.; Yuan, B.; Han, Y.; Zhang, B. Radiographic analysis of the sacral-2-alar screw trajectory. *J. Orthop. Surg. Res.* **2021**, *16*, 522. [CrossRef]
16. Denis, F.; Davis, S.; Comfort, T. Sacral fractures: An important problem. Retrospective analysis of 236 cases. *Clin. Orthop. Relat. Res.* **1988**, *227*, 67–81. [CrossRef]
17. Roy-Camille, R.; Saillant, G.; Gagna, G.; Mazel, C. Transverse fracture of the upper sacrum. Suicidal jumper's fracture. *Spine (Phila Pa 1976)* **1985**, *10*, 838–845. [CrossRef]
18. Devlin, N.J.; Brooks, R. EQ-5D and the EuroQol Group: Past, Present and Future. *Appl. Health Econ. Health Policy* **2017**, *15*, 127–137. [CrossRef]
19. Bajada, S.; Mohanty, K. Psychometric properties including reliability, validity and responsiveness of the Majeed pelvic score in patients with chronic sacroiliac joint pain. *Eur. Spine J.* **2016**, *25*, 1939–1944. [CrossRef]
20. Lin, Y.C.; Gfoehler, M.; Pandy, M.G. Quantitative evaluation of the major determinants of human gait. *J. Biomech.* **2014**, *47*, 1324–1331. [CrossRef]
21. Gordon, K.E.; Ferris, D.P.; Kuo, A.D. Metabolic and mechanical energy costs of reducing vertical center of mass movement during gait. *Arch. Phys. Med. Rehabil.* **2009**, *90*, 136–144. [CrossRef] [PubMed]
22. Kubota, M.; Uchida, K.; Kokubo, Y.; Shimada, S.; Matsuo, H.; Yayama, T.; Miyazaki, T.; Sugita, D.; Watanabe, S.; Baba, H. Post-operative gait analysis and hip muscle strength in patients with pelvic ring fracture. *Gait Posture* **2013**, *38*, 385–390. [CrossRef] [PubMed]
23. Kubota, M.; Uchida, K.; Kokubo, Y.; Shimada, S.; Matsuo, H.; Yayama, T.; Miyazaki, T.; Takeura, N.; Yoshida, A.; Baba, H. Changes in gait pattern and hip muscle strength after open reduction and internal fixation of acetabular fracture. *Arch. Phys. Med. Rehabil.* **2012**, *93*, 2015–2021. [CrossRef] [PubMed]
24. Dean, C.S.; Nadeau, J.; Strage, K.E.; Tucker, N.J.; Chambers, L.; Worster, K.; Rojas, D.; Schneider, G.; Johnson, T.; Hunt, K.; et al. Analysis of Post-operative Gait, Hip Strength, and Patient-Reported Outcomes After OTA/AO 61-B and 61-C Pelvic Ring Injuries. *J. Orthop. Trauma* **2022**, *36*, 432–438. [CrossRef]
25. Lefaivre, K.A.; Blachut, P.A.; Starr, A.J.; Slobogean, G.P.; O'Brien, P.J. Radiographic Displacement in Pelvic Ring Disruption: Reliability of 3 Previously Described Measurement Techniques. *J. Orthop. Trauma* **2014**, *28*, 160–166. [CrossRef]
26. Hashmi, S.Z.; Butler, B.; Johnson, D.; Wun, K.; Sherman, A.; Summers, H.; Stover, M. Accuracy of Radiographic Displacement Measurement in a Pelvic Ring Injury Model. *J. Am. Acad. Orthop. Surg.* **2022**, *30*, e173–e181. [CrossRef]

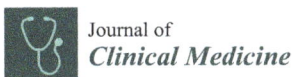

Article

Pathomechanism of Triangular Fibrocartilage Complex Injuries in Patients with Distal-Radius Fractures: A Magnetic-Resonance Imaging Study

Beom-Soo Kim *, Chul-Hyun Cho, Kyung-Jae Lee, Si-Wook Lee and Seok-Ho Byun

Department of Orthopedic Surgery, Keimyung University Dongsan Hospital, Keimyung University School of Medicine, Daegu 42601, Korea
* Correspondence: kbs090216@gmail.com; Tel.: +82-53-258-7929

Abstract: Injury to the triangular fibrocartilage complex (TFCC) is one of the most common complications following a fracture of the distal radius. In this study, an examination of TFCC injuries in patients with distal-radius fractures was conducted using magnetic-resonance imaging (MRI); the aim of the study was to analyze the prevalence of TFCC injury as well as to suggest acceptable radiologic parameters for use in prediction of the injury pattern. Fifty-eight patients with distal-radius fractures who underwent MRI prior to undergoing open-reduction surgery between April 2020 and July 2021 were included in this study. An analysis of various radiologic parameters, the fracture type, and the MRI classification of TFCC injuries was performed. Radiologic parameters were used in the evaluation of distal radioulnar joint (DRUJ), radial shortening, and the dorsal angularity of the fracture. All of the patients in this study had definite traumatic TFCC injuries. A statistical relationship was observed between the radial length gap between the intact wrist and the injured wrist, which represents relative radial shortening, and the pattern of TFCC injury. In conclusion, the shortening of the distal radius, causing peripheral soft tissue of the ulnar side to become tauter, is highly relevant with regard to the pattern of TFCC injury. However, because no data on the clinical outcome were utilized in this study, it is lacking in clinical perspective. The conduct of further studies on patients' clinical outcome will be necessary.

Keywords: distal-radius fracture; triangular fibrocartilage complex injury; magnetic-resonance-imaging study; radial length; open reduction

Citation: Kim, B.-S.; Cho, C.-H.; Lee, K.-J.; Lee, S.-W.; Byun, S.-H. Pathomechanism of Triangular Fibrocartilage Complex Injuries in Patients with Distal-Radius Fractures: A Magnetic-Resonance Imaging Study. *J. Clin. Med.* **2022**, *11*, 6168. https://doi.org/10.3390/jcm11206168

Academic Editor: Christian Carulli

Received: 5 September 2022
Accepted: 18 October 2022
Published: 19 October 2022

Publisher's Note: MDPI stays neutral with regard to jurisdictional claims in published maps and institutional affiliations.

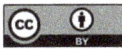

Copyright: © 2022 by the authors. Licensee MDPI, Basel, Switzerland. This article is an open access article distributed under the terms and conditions of the Creative Commons Attribution (CC BY) license (https://creativecommons.org/licenses/by/4.0/).

1. Introduction

Distal-radius fracture (DRF), one of the most common fractures occurring in elderly people, accounts for approximately 18% of fractures in patients older than 65 years [1,2]. Triangular fibrocartilage complex (TFCC) tear, the injury most associated with unstable distal-radius fractures, has been reported in 39% to 84% of cases [2,3]. This concomitant injury may contribute to the development of chronic wrist pain, decreased grip strength, and restricted motion [4].

Better visualization and diagnosis of TFCC injury can be achieved by use of arthroscopic examination; however, it is not a standardized test for use in all patients with distal-radius fractures [5,6]. Although MRI scanning is used for diagnosis of TFCC injuries, MRI testing is not performed routinely in all patients with distal-radius fractures at the time of the injury [7]. Instead, the test is recommended for patients who have symptoms related to TFCC injury after the fracture treatment has ended, which can cause a delay in the treatment of the injury.

Some studies using MRI in patients with DRF have demonstrated the prevalence of TFCC injuries; however, studies on the pathomechanism of TFCC injuries concomitant to DRF have rarely been reported [7]. According to findings from previous studies, radiologic features such as the fracture pattern, the magnitude of displacement, and the presence of an ulnar styloid fracture may be independent predictors of TFCC injuries related to DRF [2,8,9]. This study hypothesized that performing an analysis of radiologic parameters in MRI studies of patients with DRF may foster an understanding of the pathomechanism of TFCC injuries.

The purpose of this study is to a conduct radiographic examination and MRI studies in order to determine the fracture mechanism of distal-radius fracture and the prevalence and the pathomechanism of TFCC injuries concomitant to fracture.

2. Materials and Methods

Sixty-three patients underwent surgical management for the treatment of distal-radius fracture in a single fellowship-training hospital between March 2020 and July 2021. Inclusion criteria were patients who underwent open reduction and internal fixation of the fracture. Patients younger than 18 years old and those who had previously occurring arthritis of the wrist or degenerative TFCC injuries on the affected wrist were excluded. Those patients underwent MRI scanning, and five patients who refused the test were excluded, so that 58 patients were finally included in this study (Figure 1).

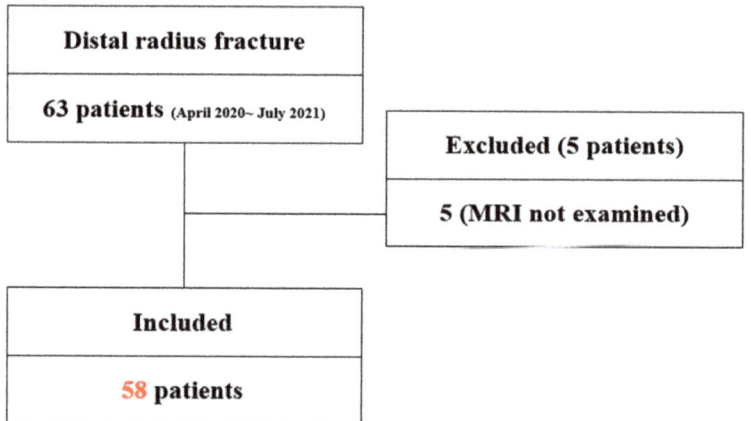

Figure 1. Patient's flow chart. Patient profiles and the groups included in the study. MRI, magnetic-resonance imaging.

An analysis of simple radiographic parameters (the radial inclination, the radial length, the distal radioulnar joint (DRUJ) gap, the sagittal/radial transition ratio, the DRUJ gap on the unaffected wrist, and the presence of a distal ulnar fracture) and patterns of TFCC injury in the MRI scan was performed by two orthopedic surgeons using the Palmar classification. Regarding the classification of fractures, the Fernandez classification and the AO/OTA classification were used in defining the mechanism of injury and the fracture pattern, respectively. Other assessments included general demographics and underlying osteoporotic disease.

A standard 4 view x-ray of the injured wrist, and AP and lateral views of the uninjured side were obtained for all patients. Measurement of the DRUJ gap distance was performed on both sides in order to better evaluate widening of the DRUJ. The DRUJ distance was defined as the maximum distance between either the volar or dorsal cortical rim of the sigmoid notch of the radius and the ulnar head. The radial translation ratio was calculated as the fraction of the DRUJ gap distance relative to the radioulnar width of the proximal fracture fragment. On the lateral X-ray, the sagittal translation was defined as the distance between the volar cortex of the radius shaft and the volar cortical margin of the distal fracture fragment. The sagittal translation ratio was calculated as the fraction of the sagittal translation to the AP width of the proximal fracture fragment [2,8].

The articular involvement of the fracture and the presence of an ulnar styloid fracture, which was then classified as a tip, middle, or base fracture each separating 1/3 of the ulnar styloid, was evaluated in this study. In addition, ulnar styloid fracture was classified as type 1,2,3 each corresponding to distal to base where the superficial horizontal fibers of the TFCC are inserted, base fracture and proximal to the base fracture, respectively [9,10].

The radial length was defined as the distance between two lines drawn perpendicular to the long axis of the radius on the AP projection from the apex of the radial styloid and the level of the ulnar aspect of the articular surface. The radial length was measured on the uninjured wrist, and the radial length gap between both sides of the wrist was obtained for the evaluation of the pure radial shortening distance (Figure 2).

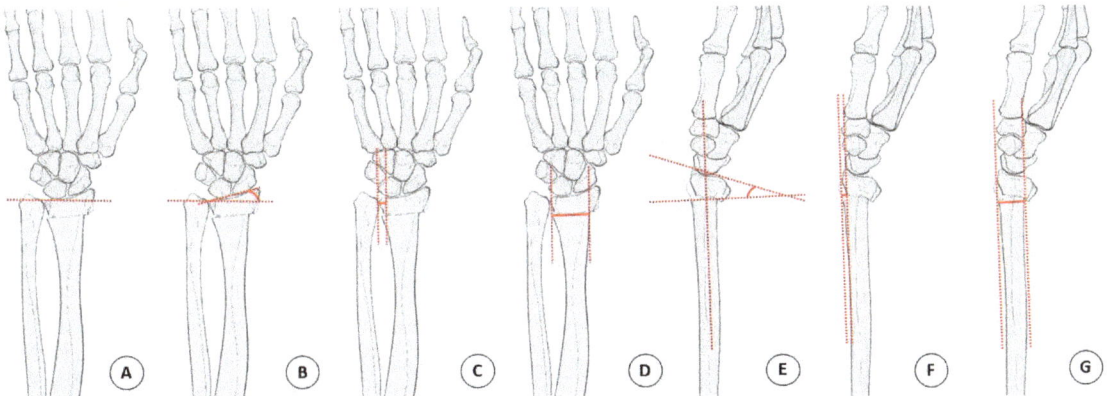

Figure 2. Radiologic parameter measurement technique. (**A**) Radial length. (**B**) Radial inclination. (**C**) DRUJ distance. (**D**) Fracture site width. (**E**) Dorsal angulation. (**F**) Sagittal translation. (**G**) Anteroposterior width. Radial translation ratio = C/D, Sagittal translation ratio = F/G. DRUJ, distal radioulnar joint.

An MRI examination of the injured wrist was performed on all patients using a 3.0 T MRI scanner (Magnetom 3.0 T, Siemens, Munich, Germany/Ingenia 3.0 T, Philip, Amsterdam, The Netherlands). Statistical analysis was performed using the SPSS statistical package (Version 22.0; IBM, Armonk, NY, USA). The Chi-square test was used for the evaluation of categorical variables, and the T-Test was used for the evaluation of continuous variables. The level of significance was set as p value < 0.05.

3. Results

The mean age of the patients was 65.21 years (range: 19–89 years; 15 male and 43 female); 15 men and 43 women were included in the study (Table 1). One patient was injured by a direct hit on the wrist, while other patients were injured by the fallen-onto-outstretched-hand (FOOSH) mechanism. According to the data from AO/OTA classification, 16 patients had A2 fractures; 8 patients had A3 fractures; 4 patients had B3 fractures; and 4, 8, and 12 patients had C1, 2, and 3 fractures, respectively (Table 2). According to the Fernandez classification, 29 patients had type I fractures, and 4, 12, and 13 patients had Type II, III, and V fractures. Twenty-six patients showed widening of the DRUJ gap compared to the unaffected wrist. Associated distal ulnar fractures were detected in 38 patients (65%). All patients in this study had a definite traumatic TFCC injury; 1A ($n = 5$), 1B ($n = 19$), 1C ($n = 33$), and 1D ($n = 1$).

Table 1. Demographic data.

Index		TFCC Pattern Relevance (p Value)
Index age (average)	65.21	>0.05
Gender (male:female ratio)	8:2	>0.05
BMI (average)	24.05	>0.05
Osteoporosis (%)	37.9	>0.05

BMI: body mass index; TFCC: triangular fibrocartilage complex.

Table 2. TFCC injury pattern.

TFCC Injury Pattern (Palmar Classification)	N
1A	5
1B	19
1C	33
1D	1

N: number; TFCC: triangular fibrocartilage complex.

No significant relationship was observed between fracture classification (AO/OTA, Fernandez) and types of TFCC injury (Palmar classification): AO/OTA, Fernandez (Table 3). Intra-articular fracture involvement, and the presence of an ulnar styloid fracture, had no significant effect on the type of TFCC injury: articular involvement ($p > 0.05$) and ulnar styloid fracture ($p > 0.05$). Type lC TFCC injuries were significant in patients with osteoporosis, compared with other groups ($p < 0.01$). Regarding age-related statistics, more Type 1C injuries were observed in significantly older patients than in younger patients ($p < 0.01$).

Table 3. Fracture classification with TFCC injury pattern.

	Palmar Classification				
	1A	1B	1C	1D	Total
AO/OTA classification					
A2	2	5	9	1	17
A3	0	5	6	0	11
B3	1	2	1	0	4
C1	1	1	2	0	4
C2	0	4	6	0	10
C3	1	2	9	0	12
Total	5	19	33	1	58
Fernandez classification					
1	2	11	15	1	29
2	1	2	1	0	4
3	1	3	8	0	12
5	1	3	9	0	13
Total	5	19	33	1	58

Fracture classification (AO/OTA, Fernandez) had no statistical significance with TFCC injury. ($p > 0.05/p > 0.05$ respectively). AO, arbeitsgemeinschaft fur osteosynthesfragen; OTA, orthopedic trauma association; and TFCC, triangular fibrocartilage complex.

For the radiologic parameters, except for the radial length gap, there was no significant difference in the type of injury (Table 4). The radial length gap between the intact wrist and the injured wrist showed significant relevance with the pattern of TFCC injury. The increased radial length gap showed relevance with type lC injuries ($p < 0.05$).

Table 4. Radiologic parameter with TFCC injury pattern.

Radiologic Parameter	Palmar Classification				p-Value
	1A	1B	1C	1D	
DRUJ gap	−0.014	0.28	0.25	0.07	>0.05
Radial length	6.69	5.25	3.14	11.9	>0.05
Radial length gap	3.53	5.04	6.27	−5.16	<0.05 *
Radial inclination	18.06	14.026	13.982	23.9	>0.05
Dorsal angulation	−2.02	5.13	7.84	−15.9	>0.05

Radiologic parameter, except radial length gap had no significant relevance with TFCC injury pattern. DRUJ, distal radioulnar joint; TFCC, triangular fibrocartilage complex; and *, statistically significant.

4. Discussion

According to a previous study, TFCC injury with an exceeding dorsal angulation of 32′ can be expected [10]. However, in this study, all TFCC injuries were detected, and dorsal angulation of more than 32′ was detected in only seven of them; there was no statistical significance with the dorsal angularity of the fracture ($p > 0.05$). In a cadaveric study, the displacement of the intact TFCC complex together with the ulnar styloid base fracture fragment was observed, while TFCC avulsion injuries were detected in patients with ulnar styloid tip fractures [10]. In this study, however, no correlation was observed between ulnar styloid fracture and patterns of TFCC injury type.

The ulnocarpal ligaments (ulnolunate and ulnotriquetral ligament) do not insert onto the ulna but are derived from the anterior part of the TFCC, and they connect the carpus to the ulnar by the palmar portion of the radioulnar ligament at its origin—the fovea. Type lC injury is defined as the distal avulsion of the carpal attachment in TFCC. Findings from this study demonstrated an association of distal avulsion with direct radial shortening, which contradicts the previously held common belief that increased dorsal angularity makes the distal avulsion force stronger. When considering the normal variance of ulnar head positioning, radial length alone in an injured wrist might not represent the degree of radial shortening. The measurement of radial length discrepancy compared with the intact wrist should be performed, and a gap of more than 6.3 mm (SD 4.7) might strongly suggest type lC TFCC injury.

As demonstrated in previous cadevaric studies, ECU subsheath (sECU), an integral part of the TFCC, provides ulnocarpal stability and appears to precede dorsal and palmar injuries. In the Bowstring phenomenon, which explains the rupture of sECU, avulsion injuries of dorsal soft tissues of the TFCC complex are manifested [10,11]. Findings from other studies have demonstrated that the dorsal angulation of distal-radius fractures causes the increased traction of palmar ligaments inserting within the foveal region, making them taut in extension and finally resulting in palmar injuries of the TFCC complex [12]. This explains the mechanism by which dorsal and palmar injuries can co-exist.

Previous studies have demonstrated an association of TFCC injuries with the degree of dorsal or volar angulation of the fracture [13,14]. In a cadaver study, sectioned TFCC resulted in increased dorsal angulation [13]. In this study, TFCC injuries were detected in all patients; however, there was no significant relationship between the degree of dorsal angularity and TFCC injury.

The conclusion of this study is that radial compression and the shortening of the distal radius causes the peripheral tear of the ulnar side, preceding the tear of the palmar ligament. The "dart-throwing motion" in the injury mechanism of the distal-radius fracture has been introduced in order to further explain this concept. The dart-throwing-motion (DTM) plane can be defined as the plane on which the functional oblique motion of the wrist occurs [15–18]. Geometric anatomical factors, ligament factors, and musculature factors have been used to explain DTM, the functional ROM that extends wrist function with radial deviation (so called radial-extension) and flexes with ulnar deviation (so called ulnar-flexion). Except for one case that had type B TFCC injury—injured caused by a direct blow from a ball—other patients were injured by the fallen-onto-outstretched-hand

(FOOSH) mechanism. When considering a dorsal angulated fracture with DTM, the axial compression force might accompany wrist extension and radial deviation not only with wrist extension, and vice versa.

Axial loading and radial deviating force during the injury mechanism of distal-radius fracture causes the shortening of the radial length. Regarding this concept of injury mechanism, the findings from this study demonstrated that radial shortening with a dorsally angulated fracture, regardless of the degree of angulation, increases tension in the soft tissue of the ulnar side, leading to the dorsal or palmar TFCC injury of the ulnar side.

Radial avulsion injury (D1) was detected in only one case, which showed a volar angulated fracture and the greatest increase in radial-length distance (Figure 3). In this case, both distal radioulnar fractures occurred; however, there was greater displacement of the distal ulnar fracture fragment, which was shortened in length, and the distal radius was volar angulated. The patient was driving at the time of injury, with her wrist in a flexed position; as the car came to a sudden stop, she suffered a direct injury from the car handle with her wrist in a flexed position. In this case, considering DTM, the direct axial force that was applied while her wrist was in a state of ulnar flexion caused greater displacement of the distal ulnar fracture. Unlike Colle's fracture mentioned above, ulnar-deviated and volar-angulating axial force decreases the tension on the palmar soft tissue of the TFCC and makes the detachment of sECU from the ulnar side more difficult, thereby transmitting the axial force to the radial avulsion of the TFCC.

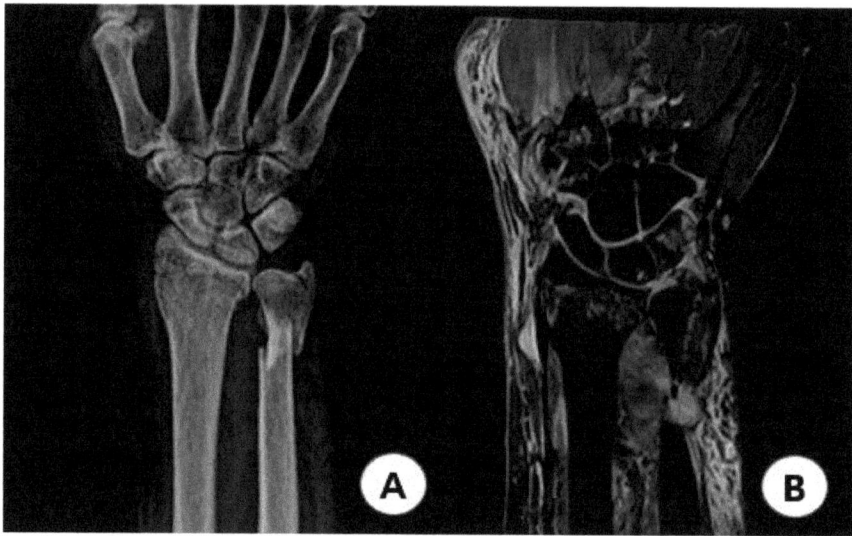

Figure 3. Type 1D injury case. Sixty-three year-old female patient injured with her wrist flexed had AO/OTA type A2 fracture with 15' volar angulation, showing 5 mm increased radial length gap (**A**), and had type 1D TFCC injury with relatively preserved peripheral and distal portion of TFCC (**B**). AO: arbeitsgemeinschaft fur osteosynthesfragen; OTA: orthopedic trauma association; and TFCC: triangular fibrocartilage complex.

MRI tests have been performed in all patients within 1–2 days after visiting our emergency center. All of the patients took MRI tests within 5 days after injury since some of them visited our clinic 2–3 days after the initial injury. Using the 3.0 T MRI scanner, examiners (two orthopedic specialists) could definitely find acute infiltration or the torn part of the TFCC, which were irrelevant with regard to joint effusion and bone-marrow edema caused by an acute injury. The final reading paper was by a radiologic specialist who also reported a definite traumatic tear in every test. This study shows a higher prevalence of TFCC injury than other studies reported, but because of the relatively poorer sensitivity of the MRI test compared to the arthroscopic examination, the possibility of false-positive results should never be overlooked [6]. Arthroscopic examination facilitates the reduction in intra-articular fracture, and it is a standard study for evaluating concomitant injury involving TFCC tear after DRF [5,6,9]. However, in this study, routine arthroscopy was not performed because patients did not fully consent to having an additional arthroscopic procedure involving general anesthesia (this procedure was not cost-efficient according to the Korean insurance system).

This study has several limitations. First, data on the clinical outcome were not utilized. TFCC injury is the most associated secondary injury after distal-radius fracture; however, because both of these injuries are mostly self-limiting or easily overcome with conservative management, including physical therapy or medication, treatment after healing of the fracture is controversial [19,20]. As demonstrated in this study, most of the patients had concomitant TFCC injuries; however, the overall outcomes after the surgery were not proven. In order to prove the clinical importance of this study, an analysis of patient outcome, such as the clinical score (VAS, Mayo, and DASH); the follow-up data; the period of symptom resolution; and the number of patients receiving additional TFCC management, including surgery, should be performed in the next study. The relatively small number of patients is another limitation of this study. Type D injury was detected in only one case, and the results cannot be supported.

5. Conclusions

In conclusion, TFCC injuries were associated with all distal-radius fracture cases in this study, regardless of types of fracture and the presence of ulnar styloid fracture. We concluded that distal radius shortening, resulting in the avulsion of TFCC ligaments, is the predominant parameter affecting the TFCC injury pattern.

Author Contributions: Conceptualization, B.-S.K.; methodology, B.-S.K.; software, S.-H.B.; validation, C.-H.C., S.-W.L.; formal analysis, S.-W.L.; investigation, S.-H.B.; resources, B.-S.K.; data curation, C.-H.C.; writing—original draft preparation, S.-H.B.; writing—review and editing, B.-S.K.; visualization, S.-W.L.; supervision, K.-J.L.; project administration, B.-S.K.; and funding acquisition, B.-S.K. All authors have read and agreed to the published version of the manuscript.

Funding: This work was supported by the research promoting grant from the Keimyung University Dongsan Medical Center in 2021.

Institutional Review Board Statement: The study was conducted according to the guidelines of the Declaration of Helsinki and approved by the Institutional Review Board (or Ethics Committee) of KMUDSH IRB (IRB No. 2021-04-124-002).

Informed Consent Statement: Informed consent was obtained from all subjects involved in the study. Written informed consent has been obtained from the patients to publish this paper.

Conflicts of Interest: The authors declare no conflict of interest.

References

1. Rundgren, J.; Bojan, A.; Mellstrand Navarro, C.; Enocson, A. Epidemiology, classification, treatment and mortality of distal radius fractures in adults: An observational study of 23,394 fractures from the national Swedish fracture register. *BMC Musculoskelet. Disord.* **2020**, *21*, 88. [CrossRef] [PubMed]
2. Fujitani, R.; Omokawa, S.; Akahane, M.; Iida, A.; Ono, H.; Tanaka, Y. Predictors of distal radioulnar joint instability in distal radius fractures. *J. Hand Surg. Am.* **2011**, *36*, 1919–1925. [CrossRef] [PubMed]
3. Im, J.; Kang, S.J.; Lee, S.J. A Comparative Study between Conservative and Surgical Treatments of Triangular Fibrocartilage Complex Injury of the Wrist with Distal Radius Fractures. *Clin. Orthop. Surg.* **2021**, *13*, 105–109. [CrossRef] [PubMed]
4. Jung, H.S.; Jung, H.S.; Baek, S.H.; Lee, J.S. How Many Screws Are Needed for Reliable Stability of Extra-articular Nonosteoporotic Distal Radius Fractures Fixed with Volar Locking Plates? *Clin. Orthop. Surg.* **2020**, *12*, 22–28. [CrossRef] [PubMed]
5. Kastenberger, T.; Kaiser, P.; Schmidle, G.; Schwendinger, P.; Gabl, M.; Arora, R. Arthroscopic assisted treatment of distal radius fractures and concomitant injuries. *Arch. Orthop. Trauma Surg.* **2020**, *140*, 623–638. [CrossRef] [PubMed]
6. Yao, J.; Fogel, N. Arthroscopy in Distal Radius Fractures: Indications and When to Do It. *Hand Clin.* **2021**, *37*, 279–291. [CrossRef] [PubMed]

7. Yan, B.; Xu, Z.; Chen, Y.; Yin, W. Prevalence of triangular fibrocartilage complex injuries in patients with distal radius fractures: A 3.0 T magnetic resonance imaging study. *J. Int. Med. Res.* **2019**, *47*, 3648–3655. [CrossRef] [PubMed]
8. Bombaci, H.; Polat, A.; Deniz, G.; Akinci, O. The value of plain X-rays in predicting TFCC injury after distal radial fractures. *J. Hand Surg. Eur. Vol.* **2008**, *33*, 322–326. [CrossRef] [PubMed]
9. Tomori, Y.; Nanno, M.; Takai, S. The Presence and the Location of an Ulnar Styloid Fracture Associated With Distal Radius Fracture Predict the Presence of Triangular Fibrocartilage Complex 1B Injury. *Arthroscopy* **2020**, *36*, 2674–2680. [CrossRef] [PubMed]
10. Scheer, J.H.; Adolfsson, L.E. Pathomechanisms of ulnar ligament lesions of the wrist in a cadaveric distal radius fracture model. *Acta Orthop.* **2011**, *82*, 360–364. [CrossRef] [PubMed]
11. Trehan, S.K.; Gould, H.P.; Meyers, K.N.; Wolfe, S.W. The Effect of Distal Radius Fracture Location on Distal Radioulnar Joint Stability: A Cadaveric Study. *J. Hand Surg. Am.* **2019**, *44*, 473–479. [CrossRef] [PubMed]
12. Scheer, J.H.; Adolfsson, L.E. Patterns of triangular fibrocartilage complex (TFCC) injury associated with severely dorsally displaced extra-articular distal radius fractures. *Injury* **2012**, *43*, 926–932. [CrossRef] [PubMed]
13. Nishiwaki, M.; Welsh, M.; Gammon, B.; Ferreira, L.M.; Johnson, J.A.; King, G.J. Distal radioulnar joint kinematics in simulated dorsally angulated distal radius fractures. *J. Hand Surg. Am.* **2014**, *39*, 656–663. [CrossRef] [PubMed]
14. Nishiwaki, M.; Welsh, M.F.; Gammon, B.; Ferreira, L.M.; Johnson, J.A.; King, G.J. Effect of Volarly Angulated Distal Radius Fractures on Forearm Rotation and Distal Radioulnar Joint Kinematics. *J. Hand Surg. Am.* **2015**, *40*, 2236–2242. [CrossRef] [PubMed]
15. Kijima, Y.; Viegas, S.F. Wrist anatomy and biomechanics. *J. Hand Surg. Am.* **2009**, *34*, 1555–1563. [CrossRef] [PubMed]
16. Moritomo, H.; Murase, T.; Goto, A.; Oka, K.; Sugamoto, K.; Yoshikawa, H. Capitate-based kinematics of the midcarpal joint during wrist radioulnar deviation: An in vivo three-dimensional motion analysis. *J. Hand Surg. Am.* **2004**, *29*, 668–675. [CrossRef] [PubMed]
17. Vardakastani, V.; Bell, H.; Mee, S.; Brigstocke, G.; Kedgley, A.E. Clinical measurement of the dart throwing motion of the wrist: Variability, accuracy and correction. *J. Hand Surg. Eur. Vol.* **2018**, *43*, 723–731. [CrossRef] [PubMed]
18. Wolfe, S.W.; Crisco, J.J.; Orr, C.M.; Marzke, M.W. The dart-throwing motion of the wrist: Is it unique to humans? *J. Hand Surg. Am.* **2006**, *31*, 1429–1437. [CrossRef] [PubMed]
19. Deniz, G.; Kose, O.; Yanik, S.; Colakoglu, T.; Tugay, A. Effect of untreated triangular fibrocartilage complex (TFCC) tears on the clinical outcome of conservatively treated distal radius fractures. *Eur. J. Orthop. Surg. Traumatol.* **2014**, *24*, 1155–1159. [CrossRef] [PubMed]
20. Kasapinova, K.; Kamiloski, V. Outcomes of surgically treated distal radius fractures associated with triangular fibrocartilage complex injury. *J. Hand Ther.* **2020**, *33*, 339–345. [CrossRef] [PubMed]

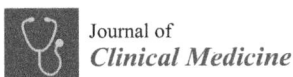

Systematic Review

The Necessity of Implant Removal after Fixation of Thoracolumbar Burst Fractures—A Systematic Review

Xing Wang [1,†], Xiang-Dong Wu [2,*,†], Yanbin Zhang [3], Zhenglin Zhu [4], Jile Jiang [3], Guanqing Li [3], Jiacheng Liu [4], Jiashen Shao [5] and Yuqing Sun [3,*]

1. Department of Spinal Surgery, Shihezi General Hospital of the Eighth Division, Shihezi 832002, China
2. Department of Orthopaedic Surgery, Beijing Jishuitan Hospital, Fourth Clinical College of Peking University, National Center for Orthopaedics, Beijing 100035, China
3. Department of Spine Surgery, Beijing Jishuitan Hospital, Fourth Clinical College of Peking University, National Center for Orthopaedics, Beijing 100035, China
4. Department of Orthopaedic Surgery, The First Affiliated Hospital of Chongqing Medical University, Chongqing 400016, China
5. Department of Orthopedics, Beijing Friendship Hospital, Capital Medical University, Beijing 100050, China
* Correspondence: wuxiangdong@jst-hosp.com.cn (X.-D.W.); syuqing2004@126.com (Y.S.)
† These authors contributed equally to this work.

Abstract: Background: Thoracolumbar burst fractures are a common traumatic vertebral fracture in the spine, and pedicle screw fixation has been widely performed as a safe and effective procedure. However, after the stabilization of the thoracolumbar burst fractures, whether or not to remove the pedicle screw implant remains controversial. This review aimed to assess the benefits and risks of pedicle screw instrument removal after fixation of thoracolumbar burst fractures. Methods: Data sources, including PubMed, EMBASE, Cochrane Library, Web of Science, Google Scholar, and Clinical trials.gov, were comprehensively searched. All types of human studies that reported the benefits and risks of implant removal after thoracolumbar burst fractures, were selected for inclusion. Clinical outcomes after implant removal were collected for further evaluation. Results: A total of 4051 papers were retrieved, of which 35 studies were eligible for inclusion in the review, including four case reports, four case series, and 27 observational studies. The possible risks of pedicle screw removal after fixation of thoracolumbar burst fractures include the progression of the kyphotic deformity and surgical complications (e.g., surgical site infection, neurovascular injury, worsening pain, revision surgery), while the potential benefits of pedicle screw removal mainly include improved segmental range of motion and alleviated pain and disability. Therefore, the potential benefits and possible risks should be weighed to support patient-specific clinical decision-making about the removal of pedicle screws after the successful fusion of thoracolumbar burst fractures. Conclusions: There was conflicting evidence regarding the benefits and harms of implant removal after successful fixation of thoracolumbar burst fractures, and the current literature does not support the general recommendation for removal of the pedicle screw instruments, which may expose the patients to unnecessary complications and costs. Both surgeons and patients should be aware of the indications and have appropriate expectations of the benefits and risks of implant removal. The decision to remove the implant or not should be made individually and cautiously by the surgeon in consultation with the patient. Further studies are warranted to clarify this issue. Level of evidence: level 1.

Keywords: thoracolumbar burst fracture; implant; pedicle screw; removal; kyphosis; complications; pain

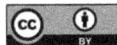

1. Introduction

A new spinal fracture occurs every 22 s worldwide [1]. As a mechanical transition junction between the relatively rigid thoracic and the more flexible lumbar spine, the thoracolumbar region is the most common site of fracture to the spine, and burst fractures of the thoracolumbar spine account for approximately 20–50% of such injuries [2,3]. Though common, the management of thoracolumbar burst fractures presents several clinical challenges, which mainly include surgical indications (surgery vs. non-surgery), surgical approach (anterior vs. posterior; traditional open approach vs. minimally invasive percutaneous approach), and surgical options (e.g., short segment fixation vs. long segment fixation, fusion vs. non-fusion) [4–12]. In any case, pedicle screw fixation has been well established as a standard procedure for the treatment of unstable thoracolumbar burst fractures that aims to establish immediate stability and rapid restoration of spinal alignment, prevent neurologic deterioration, minimize pain, and protect the spinal cord from further neurological injury [13–16].

After fracture consolidation has been achieved, there is another considerable controversy related to the pedicle screw instrument removal. So far, several indications have gained wide acceptance for implant removal after spinal surgery, including infection, pedicle screw misplacement, periprosthetic fracture, implant loosening, implant failure, instrumentation protrusion and local irritation, and growth disturbance [17–19]. However, the indications, potential benefits, and possible risks for implant removal in successful fracture-healing patients remain controversial [18]. Possible concerns of in situ implants are thought to be reduced range of motion, potential back pain due to mechanical irritation, micromotion, implant prominence and irritation, disc degeneration, facet arthrosis, fretting corrosion, allergic reaction, low-grade infection, stress shielding-related osteopenia, and stress concentration at the adjacent segment [17–24]. Pedicle screw removal might be a beneficial and cost-effective procedure because it can alleviate pain and discomfort, improve the segmental motion angle, restore flexibility, and enhance functional outcomes [25,26]. However, pedicle screw implants should not be considered dispensable when fracture consolidation is present, and implant removal should, by no means, be considered a benign and harmless procedure. On the contrary, implant removal requires a second operative procedure, which is accompanied by risks such as surgical site infection, neurovascular injury, significant loss of segmental kyphosis correction, worsened back pain, and re-fracture [25,26].

To date, there remains a paucity of expert consensus or clinical practice guidelines relating to implant removal after thoracolumbar burst fractures [18]. Thus, we undertook a systematic review to investigate the potential benefit-to-risk ratio and provide up-to-date evidence.

2. Materials and Methods

This systematic review was conducted following the recommendation of the *Cochrane Handbook for Systematic Reviews of Interventions* [27] and is reported in compliance with the *Preferred Reporting Items for Systematic Reviews and Meta-Analyses* (PRISMA) guidelines [28].

2.1. Data Sources

Electronic databases, including PubMed, EMBASE, Cochrane Library, Web of Science, Google Scholar, and Clinical Trials.gov, were searched from inception to November 2022. Search terms included controlled terms from Medical Subject Headings (MeSH) in PubMed, EMtree in EMBASE.com, corresponding keywords, and free text terms. The search terms included those related to "Thoracolumbar fracture", "Pedicle screw", and "Removal". The complete search strategy is presented in the electronic Supplementary Material Table S1. No language, publication status, or other search restriction was imposed. In addition, we checked the reference lists from all retrieved studies and meta-analyses or systematic reviews already published to ensure that all studies could be identified.

2.2. Eligibility Criteria

Published studies were included if they met the following inclusion criteria:

(i) **Participants**: adult patients who underwent internal fixation for thoracolumbar burst fractures;
(ii) **Intervention** and/or **comparison**: removal or retention of the pedicle screw instrument after successful fixation of thoracolumbar burst fractures;
(iii) **Outcomes**: clinical outcomes related to the benefits or harms of implant removal were considered. The primary outcomes were local kyphosis deformity after implant removal and pain intensity after implant removal. Secondary outcomes included improvement of segmental motion angle and removal-related complications;
(iv) **Study type**: All types of studies that reported the benefits and risks of implant removal after thoracolumbar burst fractures were considered for inclusion, including but not limited to case reports and case series, cohort studies, case–control studies, cross-over studies, and randomized controlled trials.

2.3. Study Selection

Identified papers from each of the databases were imported into Endnote reference management software X9 (Clarivate Analytics). Two authors independently removed the duplicates, examined the titles and reviewed the abstracts for relevance, and then sorted the remaining records for "inclusion", "exclusion", or "potentially relevant". The full-text articles of eligible records rated "potentially relevant" were obtained, reviewed, and rated independently by the two reviewers. Any discrepancies were resolved by discussion between the authors.

2.4. Data Extraction

The data were extracted using a standardized data extraction form and entered into an excel sheet (Excel, Microsoft Corporation, WA, USA). The following study details were extracted where possible from included studies: first author, publication year, region, publication journal, type of study, year of study, sample size, participant demographic details, thoracolumbar fracture level, surgical approach, segmental fixation, time to implant removal, cause of implant removal, and clinical outcomes after implant removal. Data from the research were compared, and disagreements were resolved by consensus among researchers.

2.5. Quality Assessment

The Newcastle–Ottawa Scale (NOS) was used to assess the quality of non-randomized studies [29]. The quality of included studies was evaluated in the following three major components: selection of the study group (0–4 points); quality of the adjustment for confounding (0–2 points); and assessment of the outcome of interest in the cohorts (0–3 points). A higher score represented better methodological quality.

2.6. Statistical Analysis

Meta-analysis was performed only when there were at least three contrasts available for data synthesis. Risk ratios (RRs) with 95% confidence intervals (CIs) were calculated for dichotomous data, and the mean difference (MD) or standardized mean difference (SMD) along with corresponding 95% CIs were calculated for continuous outcomes. Heterogeneity was assessed using the Cochran Q statistic ($p < 0.1$) and measured with the I^2 statistic. Meta-analyses were conducted using a random-effects model regardless of heterogeneity. Two-sided $p < 0.05$ was considered statistically significant. We used Stata version 15 (Stata Corporation, College Station, TX, USA) for data analyses.

3. Results

3.1. Study Selection

The initial search yielded 4051 records; after removing 1558 duplicates, 2493 articles were screened using the title and/or abstract. Of these, 2424 records were eliminated for being irrelevant to our analysis by screening titles and abstracts. The full texts of the remaining 69 articles were retrieved for further assessment. Finally, 35 studies were included in the systematic review [30–64]. Figure 1 displays a flow diagram that shows the reasons for exclusion at each stage of the selection process.

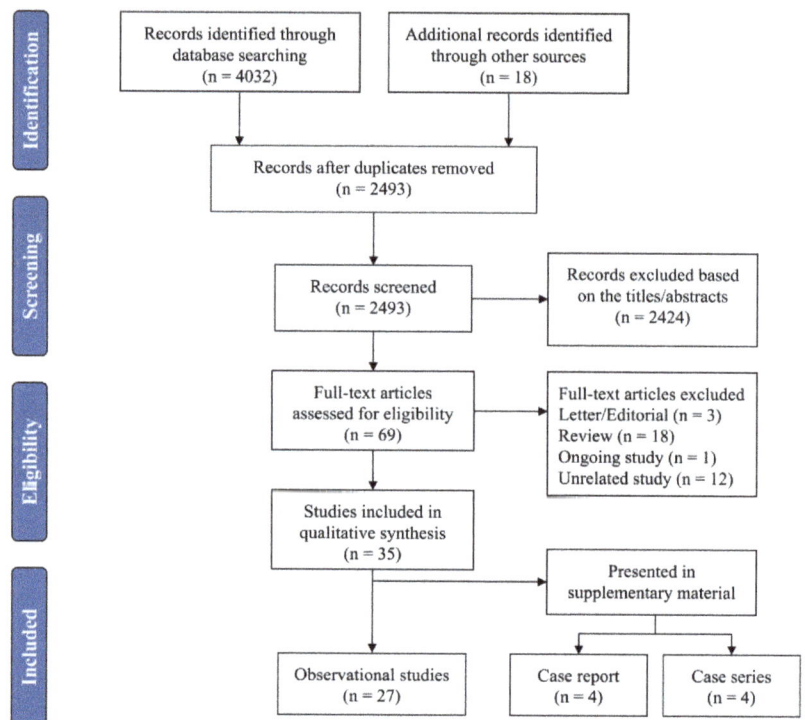

Figure 1. PRISMA flow diagram.

3.2. Study Characteristics

The main characteristics of the included observational studies are presented in Table 1, and the main characteristics of the included case reports and case series are shown in Supplementary Material Table S2. In total, four case reports [30–33], four case series [34–37], 21 retrospective cohort studies [38–45,47–49,52,53,55–58,60,61,63,64], three retrospective case-control studies [46,51,62], and three prospective cohort studies [50,54,59] were included in this systematic review. These studies were published between 1997 and 2022 [30–64]. Among the included studies, 25 were from Asia [33–36,39,40,42–50,52,54–56,60,61,63,64], six were from Europe [31,32,37,41,51,53], and four from North America [30,38,59,62]. Except for Xu et al. [64], which included patients aged over 65 years, other trials were of adult patients [30–63]. The fracture level, surgical management, fixation methods, time to implant removal, the reason for implant removal, and duration of follow-up were also quite different among the studies. The more-detailed characteristics of the included observational studies are listed in Table 2, and other detailed characteristics of included case reports and case series are summarized in Supplementary Material Table S3.

Table 1. Baseline characteristics of the included observational studies.

First Author	Publication Year	Region	Journal	Type of Study	Study Dates	No. of Patients	Age (year)	Gender	Fracture Level	Approach
Knop et al. [38]	2001	USA	Spine	Retrospective Cohort	January 1989–July 1992	76 patients	34 (range 15–63)	26F:30M	Thoracolumbar fractures	Posterior Open
Song et al. [39]	2007	South Korea	Journal of the Korean Orthopaedic Association	Retrospective Cohort	—	58 patients	—	—	Thoracolumbar burst fractures	Posterior approach
Xu et al. [40]	2009	China	Orthopaedic Surgery	Retrospective Cohort	February 1987–June 1995	89 patients	39.1 (range 21–59)	16F:52 M	Thoracolumbar fractures	Posterior approach
Stavridis et al. [41]	2010	Germany	Archives of Orthopaedic and Trauma Surgery	Retrospective Cohort	—	57 patients	46.5 (range 21–84)	28F:29M	Thoracolumbar spine	Posterior approach
Yang et al. [42]	2011	China	Global Spine Journal	Retrospective Cohort	1998–2005	64 patients	42.1 (range 18–70)	24F:40M	Thoracolumbar burst fractures	Posterior Open
Wang et al. [43]	2013	China	European Spine Journal	Retrospective Cohort	July 2007–November 2009	26 patients	39.6 ± 10.3 (range 21–54)	7F:19M	Thoracolumbar burst fractures	Posterior percutaneous
Kim et al. [44]	2014	South Korea	Journal of Korean Neurosurgical Society	Retrospective Cohort	May 2007–January 2011	44 patients	52.5	6F:10M	Thoracolumbar burst fractures	Posterior percutaneous
Ko et al. [45]	2014	South Korea	Journal of Spinal Disorders and Techniques	Retrospective Cohort	September 2003–December 2009	62 patients	38.5 (range 16–54)	29F:31M	Thoracolumbar and lumbar unstable burst fracture	Posterior Open
Jeon et al. [46]	2015	South Korea	Spine	Case–Control	June 2008–October 2011	45 patients	39.7 (range 18–62)	20F:25M	Thoracolumbar burst fractures	Posterior Open
Aono et al. [47]	2016	Japan	Injury	Retrospective Cohort	September 2006–July 2012	27 patients	43 (range 20–66)	8F:19M	Thoracolumbar burst fractures	Posterior Open
Chen et al. [48]	2016	China	International Orthopaedics	Retrospective Cohort	January 2008–December 2013	122 patients	38	49F:73M	Thoracolumbar burst fracture	Posterior Open
Chou et al. [49]	2016	Taiwan	The Bone & Joint Journal	Retrospective Cohort	June 1996–May 2012	69 patients	45.3 ± 10.2 (range 34–56)	25F:44M	burst thoracolumbar or lumbar fracture	Posterior Open
Aono et al. [50]	2017	Japan	The Spine Journal	Prospective Cohort	September 2006–October 2013	62 patients	40 (range13–69)	20F:42M	Thoracolumbar burst fracture	Posterior Open

Table 1. Cont.

First Author	Publication Year	Region	Journal	Type of Study	Study Dates	No. of Patients	Age (year)	Gender	Fracture Level	Approach
Hoppe et al. [51]	2017	Switzerland	Global Spine Journal	Retrospective Case-control	2000–2013	59 patients	41.7 ± 15.4	12F:17M	Thoracolumbar fractures	Posterior Open
Lee et al. [52]	2017	South Korea	Spine	Retrospective Cohort	February 2009–May 2012	88 patients	40.2 ± 12.8	23F:22M	Thoracolumbar burst fractures	Posterior Open
Smits et al. [53]	2017	The Netherlands	European Spine Journal	Retrospective Cohort	2003–2015	102 patients	38 (range 18–78)	47F:55M	Thoracolumbar fractures	Posterior open or combined anterior and posterior stabilization
Aono et al. [54]	2019	Japan	Journal of Clinical Neuroscience	Prospective Cohort	September 2006–May 2016	76 patients	40 (range 13–69)	24F:52M	Thoracolumbar burst fractures	Posterior Open
Oh et al. [55]	2019	South Korea	Clinics in Orthopedic Surgery	Retrospective Cohort	March 2011–October 2017	30 patients	41.4 ± 16.0 (range 16–73)	14F:16M	Thoracolumbar fractures	Posterior percutaneous
Chen et al. [56]	2020	China	World Neurosurgery	Retrospective Cohort	February 2008–December 2014	87 patients	41.3 ± 8.2 (range 17–60)	28F:56M	Thoracolumbar burst fractures	Posterior Open
Hou et al. [57]	2020	China	Beijing Da Xue Xue Bao Yi Xue Ban	Retrospective Cohort	January 2010–December 2017	144 patients	39.1 ± 13.2	70F:74M	Thoracolumbar burst fractures	Posterior Open
Ko et al. [58]	2020	South Korea	Medicine	Retrospective Cohort	March 2004–January 2007	27 patients	34.8 (range 18–49)	11F:8M	Thoracolumbar burst fractures	Posterior Open
Manson et al. [59]	2020	Canada	Advances in Orthopedics	Prospective Cohort	24-month–8 years	32 patients	38.3 (range 18–61)	8F:24M	Thoracolumbar fractures	Posterior percutaneous
Sasagawa et al. [60]	2021	Japan	Asian Journal of Neurosurgery	Retrospective Cohort	—	24 patients	43.9 ± 12.3 (range 25–64)	4F:20M	Thoracolumbar fractures	Posterior percutaneous
Hirahata et al. [61]	2022	Japan	BMC Musculoskeletal Disorders	Retrospective Cohort	December 2008–June 2016	59 patients	38 (range 17–68)	31F:28M	Thoracolumbar burst fractures	Posterior open
Kenfack et al. [62]	2022	USA	Global Spine Journal	Retrospective Case-control	2012–2017	58 patients	—	15F:43M	Thoracolumbar fractures	Posterior percutaneous
Wu et al. [63]	2022	China	World Neurosurgery	Retrospective Cohort	2018–2020	81 patients	43	21F:29M	Thoracolumbar fractures	Posterior open
Xu et al. [64]	2022	China	Frontiers in Surgery	Retrospective Cohort	August 2011–August 2018	96 patients	69.4 (range 65–77)	51F:45M	Thoracolumbar fractures	Posterior percutaneous or open

Abbreviations: F, female; M, male; —, Not Reported.

Table 2. Reported clinical outcomes in the observational studies.

Study	Fixation	Time to Implant Removal	Pre-Removal	Segmental Motion Angle	Post-Removal Pain	Post-Removal Kyphosis Deformity	Removal Complications	Follow-Up Period
Knop et al. [38] 2001	Short segment fixation	15 (range 7–35) months	—	Improved	—	Average correction loss 10.1°	A late deep wound infection 9 months after removal	25 (range 3–48) months
Song et al. [39] 2007	Fixation with fusion	—	Symptomatic (pain and discomfort)	—	VAS decreased from 6.5 to 3.2	Average correction loss 3.7°	Anterior height of the fractured vertebral body decreased by 1.5% after removal	—
Xu et al. [40] 2009	Short segment fixation	13.2 (range 8–24) months	8 patients with implant failure	—	—	Average correction loss 5.8°	5 patients had local kyphosis of >20° and more back pain, 1 patient underwent revision surgery	8 (range 5–13) years
Stavridis et al. [41] 2010	—	—	Symptomatic (implant-associated pain)	—	VAS from 62 to 48	—	5 of 57 patients (8.8%) had complications, (1 infection, 1 hematoma, 1 transient brachial plexus paresis, 2 immediate postoperative pain)	—
Yang et al. [42] 2011	Short segment fixation without fusion	9–12 months	4 patients with implant failure	—	—	Average correction loss 6.9°	—	—
Wang et al. [43] 2013	Short segment fixation without fusion	9–12 months	—	—	—	No significant kyphosis of the fracture area was diagnosed	The Pfirrmann grade of degenerative discs adjacent to the cranial fractured endplates deteriorated from 2.1 to 3.4 after implant removal	23.5 (15–36) months
Kim et al. [44] 2014	Short segment fixation without fusion	12 months	Symptomatic (pain)	Marked improvement in ROM	Significant pain relief	—	Some vertebral height loss after implant removal	11.8 months
Ko et al. [45] 2014	Short segment fixation without fusion	10 (8–14) months	Selected patients	Improved	—	Average correction loss 1.2° ± 1.63°	Correction loss after removal was due to loss of disk height and/or disk degeneration after implant removal	38 (range 15–79) months
Jeon et al. [46] 2015	Long segment fixation with fusion	18.3 ± 17.6 months	Asymptomatic	From 1.6° ± 1.5° to 5.9° ± 4.1°	From 3.8 ± 2.1 to 2.1 ± 1.7	No significant change	3 cases of superficial surgical site infection	2 years
Aono et al. [47] 2016	Short segment fixation without fusion	50 (range 24–84) months	Asymptomatic (except 1 implant failure)	Mean range of motion 8°	10 patients had increasing back pain	Average correction loss 7.5°	Postoperative correction loss occurred due to disc degeneration, especially after implant removal	2 years
Chen et al. [48] 2016	Short segment fixation without fusion	12 months	—	—	—	Average correction loss 6.3°	Kyphosis recurrence 43.4% (53 of 122 patients)	25 months
Chou et al. [49] 2016	Short segment fixation without fusion	10.3 (8–13) months	—	3.8° ± 1.2° (2°–7°)	Significant pain relief, from 6.6 ± 1.6 to 1.7 ± 0.7	Average correction loss 16.6° ± 4.9° (range 6°–26°)	Progressive loss of injured disc height may play an important role in progressive kyphosis	12 months
Aono et al. [50] 2017	Short segment fixation without fusion	12 months	Asymptomatic (except 1 implant failure)	—	—	Average correction loss 9.2° ± 4.0°	Fractured vertebral body was maintained, kyphotic deformity occurred because of a loss of disc height after implant removal	12 months
Hoppe et al. [51] 2017	Short segment fixation with fusion	9.8 ± 4.5 months	Asymptomatic	—	—	Average correction loss 6.0° ± 4.2° (range 0°–16°)	—	12.8 (range 11–14) months

111

Table 2. Cont.

Study	Fixation	Time to Implant Removal	Pre-Removal	Segmental Motion Angle	Post-Removal Pain	Post-Removal Kyphosis Deformity	Removal Complications	Follow-Up Period
Lee et al. [52] 2017	Long segment fixation with fusion	18.7 ± 7.6 months	Asymptomatic	—	—	—	1 superficial wound infection	3 years
Smits et al. [53] 2017	Fixation without fusion	median12 (IQR 10–14) months	Most asymptomatic	—	Majority relief, and minority worse	Average correction loss 4.9°	8 cases of complications (3 superficial wound infection, 2 deep wound infection, 1 instability after removal, 1 bleeding, 1 pneumonia)	>1 year
Aono et al. [54] 2019	Short segment fixation without fusion	12 months	Asymptomatic	—	—	Average correction loss 6.9°	Postoperative kyphotic change was related to disc level, not to the fractured vertebra	>1 year
Oh et al. [55] 2019	Short segment fixation without fusion	12.8 months	—	Slight improvement after implant removal, mean ROM 4.1° considered to be motionless	—	Average correction loss 3.9° ± 7.3°	Two cases of screw breakage were observed when implants were removed	5.5 months
Chen et al. [56] 2020	Short segment fixation	12 months	—	ODI from 15.9 ± 6.4 to 8.4 ± 4.6	VAS from 2.9 ± 1.3 to 1.2 ± 0.8	Average correction loss 1.5° ± 0.8°	—	>1 year
Hou et al. [57] 2020	Short segment fixation without fusion	12–18 months	Asymptomatic	—	—	Recurrent kyphosis, 92/144 (63.9%)	—	>6 months
Ko et al. [58] 2020	Short segment fixation without fusion	12.2 (range 8–15) months	Asymptomatic	Segmental motion 10.43° ± 3.32°	—	Average correction loss 16.78°	Statistically significant improvement in quality of life over time, with SF-36 56.58 ± 21.56 to 76.73 ± 17.24	>10 year
Manson et al. [59] 2020	Fixation without fusion	16–45 months	Instrumentation prominent or loosening, causing discomfort/pain	Minimal disability after removal, ODI score from 27 to 14	Dropped from moderate to mild/NRS score from 5 to 3	—	—	24 months
Sasagawa et al. [60] 2021	Fixation without fusion	14.4 ± 4.9 (range 5–27) months	—	4 of 21 patients reported improved range of motion	12 of 21 patients reported reduced back pain or discomfort	Average correction loss 9.55°	Disc degeneration happened in 16 of 24 patients	29.1 ± 17.3 (range 3–59) months
Hirahata et al. [61] 2022	Fixation without fusion	16 months	—	—	—	Kyphotic deformity (kyphotic angle >25°) was found in 17 cases (29%)	Loss of correction (kyphotic angle >15°) was found in 35 cases (59%)	15 months
Kenfack et al. [62] 2022	Fixation without fusion	—	—	No significant improvement	—	—	Patient status was not worse after implant removal	—
Wu et al. [63] 2022	Fixation without fusion	8.8–67.1 months	When bone fusion was confirmed on CT	Mean ODI declined significantly	VAS for back pain decreased significantly	Correction loss range 5.0°–8.6°	—	9.1 ± 5.7 months
Xu et al. [64] 2022	Short segment fixation without fusion	16.8 (range 12–34) months	When bony union of the fractured vertebrae was confirmed	ODI from 8.7 ± 10.7 to 8.3 ± 11.0	VAS for back pain from 1.1 ± 1.4 to 1.2 ± 1.6	Cobb angle increased from 9.6° ± 14.1° to 11.4° ± 14.4°	—	33.4 months

Abbreviations: CT, Computed Tomography; NRS, Numeric Rating Scale; ODI, Oswestry Disability Index; ROM, Range of Motion; SF-36, Short Form 36; VAS, Visual Analogue Scale; —, Not Reported.

3.3. Risk of Bias

The pre-planned risk of bias was not assessed during this systematic review. Due to the present lack of high-quality evidence, case reports and case series studies were predetermined to be included to provide related information on our topic. Even if we also included retrospective cohort studies, retrospective case–control studies, and prospective cohort studies, the quality of the observational studies was not assessed due to the inherent biases associated with these study designs and the lack of a control group in many studies.

In addition, the pre-defined meta-analyses were unfeasible due to insufficient data for these clinical outcomes and considerable clinical heterogeneity and variations in outcome measures.

3.4. Primary Outcomes

3.4.1. LOCAL Kyphosis Deformity after Implant Removal

Among the 27 observational studies, 20 studies reported varying degrees of sagittal correction loss or local kyphosis deformity, while two studies [43,46] reported no significant kyphosis of the fracture area. In detail, six studies reported average correction loss of less than 5° [39,45,53,55,56,64], nine studies reported 5°–10° average correction loss [40,42,47,48,50,51,54,56,60,63], three studies reported more than 10° average correction loss [38,49,58], and two studies reported 63.9% and 29% local kyphotic deformity after implant removal [57,61].

3.4.2. Pain Intensity after Implant Removal

Of the 27 observational studies, nine [39,41,44,46,49,53,56,59,63] reported significant pain relief after implant removal; of these, four studies [39,41,44,59] reported the decision to remove the pedicle screw instrument due to implant-associated symptoms such as pain or discomfort, while in three studies [46,53,59] the patients were asymptomatic before implant removal. One retrospective cohort study [47] found that 10 of 27 patients had increasing back pain after implant removal, while in another retrospective cohort study [60], 12 of 21 patients reported reduced back pain or discomfort after surgery. In addition, one study [64] found no significant changes after implant removal.

3.5. Secondary Outcomes

3.5.1. Improvement of Segmental Motion Angle

Among the observational studies, six [38,44–47,58] reported improvement after implant removal, three [56,59,63] reported decreased Oswestry Disability Index (ODI) scores, and one [60] reported four of 21 patients had improved range of motion. In contrast, four studies [49,55,62,64] demonstrated no or slight improvement after implant removal but the segmental motion angle was considered to be motionless.

3.5.2. Removal-Related Complications

One case report [30] reported inadvertent screw migration into the retroperitoneal space, while one case series [37] reported that pedicular screws fractured and the threaded parts of the screws were, therefore, left in 1 patient.

For the 27 observational studies, five [38,46,51–53] reported wound infection after implant removal, Two studies [39,44] reported vertebral height loss after implant removal, seven [43,45,47,49,50,54,60] reported disc degeneration and progressive loss of injured disc height, and one [40] reported revision surgery after implant removal.

4. Discussion

4.1. Principal Findings

This systematic review showed that dozens of studies focused on the benefits and risks of implant removal after fixation of thoracolumbar burst fractures, and local kyphosis deformity was the most prevalent and most important sequelae after implant removal. However, some studies further confirmed reduced pain intensity and improved segmental motion angle after implant removal. In addition, implant removal-associated complications were not uncommon.

4.2. Comparison with Previous Studies

Kweh et al. published a systematic review and meta-analysis addressing a similar topic [65]. This study eventually included 13 articles for qualitative synthesis and six studies for quantitative synthesis. They found no statistically significant difference in sagittal correction loss between implant retention and removal cohorts, and suggested significantly improved pain intensity and ODI scores. They concluded that planned implant removal results in superior functional outcomes without significant differences in kyphotic angle correction loss compared to implant retention in younger patients with thoracolumbar burst fractures who undergo posterior surgical stabilization. In comparison, we included more types of studies to fully elaborate on this clinical dilemma. Although we did not perform a meta-analysis mainly due to the significant clinical heterogeneity among studies, we found similar benefits but also highlighted the potential risks. We further revealed conflicting evidence regarding the management of thoracolumbar burst fractures.

4.3. Implication for Clinical Practice

Although implant removal accounts for almost one-third of all elective operations in orthopedics, there remains an ongoing debate concerning the justification for such procedures [32]. The thoracolumbar junction is a transitional zone that constitutes the relatively fixed kyphotic thoracic area and the mobile lordotic lumbar region; therefore, it is a vulnerable region for injury. In theory, when natural bone healing and consolidation of fractured vertebrae has occurred, implant removal should allow complete motion segment preservation, but it is hard to decide for the thoracolumbar junction.

4.3.1. Kyphosis Recurrence

Kyphosis recurrence after implant removal is not uncommon (Table 2 and Supplementary Material Table S3). Previous studies have suggested that kyphotic recurrence is inevitable during the medium- to long-term period, regardless of the pedicle screw fixation with or without fusion, and the process of kyphotic recurrence may be accelerated after removal of the pedicle screw instrument, which has been reported in case reports and case series, and some of the observational studies [50,56]. However, there remains a lack of robust clinical evidence and long-term follow-up data, and our systematic review found that currently conflicting data was more present, highlighting this clinical dilemma.

In addition, these studies also investigated the mechanism of sagittal correction loss after implant removal. Some studies [39,44] have implicated that failure to support the anterior spinal column and vertebra collapse after implant removal lead to eventual loss of correction; however, more recent studies [38,46,51–53] have found that intervertebral disc collapse and loss of disc height are the main factors contributing to postoperative kyphosis in patients with thoracolumbar burst fracture, no matter with or without vertebroplasty. Patients with incomplete and complete thoracolumbar burst fractures always suffer severely injured endplates and discs, so post-traumatic disc degeneration and height loss when loaded after implant removal are unavoidable. Thus, a mono-segmental fusion is better indicated in cases of expected disc injury to prevent secondary loss of reduction resulting from the collapse of the disc space, especially in younger patients. Removal of the implants may, therefore, not be necessary.

The relatively high incidence of kyphosis recurrence after implant removal may be caused by various factors. The surgical intervention for thoracolumbar burst fracture aims to restore stability, prevent neurological deterioration, attain canal clearance, prevent kyphosis, and provide rapid pain relief. Therefore, sufficient stability is important to avoid postoperative loss of segmental kyphosis correction, regardless of whether fusion is performed. Although the pedicle screw instrument is only to provide temporary fixation of the unstable spine and permanent restoration of spinal stability through achieving a solid fusion as the primary purpose, the pedicle screw instrument may still play an important role in maintaining the reduction, offering rigid fixation, and enhance bony union or fusion after bone healing. A previous study also suggested that the severity of the initial trauma also predicts the loss of correction after implant removal: the more severe the preoperative collapse of the fractured vertebral body is, the higher loss of correction after implant removal has to be expected [51]. In addition, other factors, such as the integrity of the posterior ligamentous complex, are also crucial, and implant removal in patients with non-healing of the posterior ligamentous complex would also induce instability and progressive kyphosis [53,56,66].

4.3.2. Segmental Range of Motion

Improvement of the segmental range of motion has been recognized as one of the major benefits of implant removal, especially in patients who received pedicle screw fixation without fusion. Several previous studies have confirmed the advantages of implant removal for the preservation of segmental motion, which can further alleviate pain and disability [38,44–47,58] and lead to decreases in the pain intensity score and ODI score [39,41,44,56,59,63]. Therefore, these clinical benefits after implant removal are measurable and demonstrate that a subgroup of patients would benefit from implant removal, especially when there was no disastrous kyphosis deformity recurrence. Nonetheless, we should also realize that the actual mobility of the segment has possible implications—both positive and negative. The improved range of motion of the fractured segment in the thoracolumbar junction would unload the stress on the adjacent segments but put stress on the fractured vertebra and nearby discs. Hence, the improved segmental range of motion also means an unstable status after implant removal, with a potential risk of recurrent kyphosis deformity induced by destabilization after implant removal [37].

4.4. Decision-Making

Removing the pedicle screw instrument after posterior fixation of thoracolumbar burst fractures can effectively restore flexibility and relieve pain, but can also result in the progression of kyphosis. Moreover, it is impossible to predict the recurrence of kyphotic deformity before implant removal, and extra revision surgery might be needed later if patients have severe back pain due to severe kyphotic deformity. Thus, careful consideration should be made before removing the implant.

In most symptomatic cases, the patient is the initiator of pedicle screw removal. Many patients with persistent symptoms tend to blame the metallic implants; they often insist on implant removal and believe this will alleviate their symptoms [67,68]. However, in clinical practice, even in patients who have reported implant-related pain, removing the implant does not guarantee pain relief and may be associated with further complications (such as infection, re-fracture, and nerve damage) and worsening pain [31,32,37,41]. Therefore, patients should be notified of indications for implant removal and understand the uncertainty of expected benefits, potential complications, and inherent risks. On the contrary, implant retention would reduce costs and alleviate exposure to further surgery, but patients should also be informed of the possibility of screw breakage.

Surgeons are the decision-makers of implant removal [18,67]. The decision of implant removal should be predetermined as early as the initial treatment of the thoracolumbar burst fractures and dynamically adjusted according to the patient's clinical status (Figure 2). Careful preoperative evaluation and consideration should be made before removing the implant. First of all, surgeons should review details of the primary thoracolumbar burst fractures, such as the mechanism of injury, the morphology, and classification of the burst fractures, and learn about the first surgical management. Second, surgeons need to assess the fusion of the burst fractures, which is critical but challenging, and even intra-operative exploration demonstrates that a solid fusion cannot promise desired outcomes [67]. Next, for symptomatic patients, surgeons should try to figure out to what extent the patient's pain and discomfort are associated with the pedicle screw instrument, and how much pain relief can be expected from implant removal [69]. For example, postoperative pain may be attributed to instability, root pain, adjacent-level pathology, and factors related to the implant. Very often, the exact cause of post-instrumented pain remains difficult to determine. Finally, communication with patients is essential and crucial than ever before [41]. Patients should be informed thoroughly about the unpredictable outcomes of implant removal to avoid excessively high expectations [41]. Moreover, detailed preoperative evaluation before implant removal is also indispensable. For instance, a CT scan before implant removal would be beneficial for confirmation of posterolateral fusion and preoperative measurement of the bone mineral density of the fractured vertebral body and adjacent vertebral bodies to evaluate the risk of compression fracture after implant removal [31,32]. Based on these careful preoperative clinical evaluations and detailed communication, a decision to remove or retain the implants could be made. The timing of the removal of the implant remains an open question.

4.5. Call for Future Studies

The currently available evidence for removing or retaining the pedicle screw instrument in thoracolumbar burst fractures is heterogeneous, limited, and insufficient. Thus, more prospective cohort studies and clinical trials with long-term follow-ups are strongly warranted to provide additional details about the advantages and disadvantages of each option, which would help mitigate the trade-off between the benefits and harms of different treatment options. Second, there is a desperate need to explore the biological mechanisms and clinical determinants of symptomatic and asymptomatic implants, as well as the risk factors and predictive parameters for the recurrence of kyphotic deformity, which will contribute to developing clinical decision rules that may determine which patient subgroup will benefit most from implant removal and which patient subgroup will face more risks [69,70]. Next, future studies should compare the same types of fractures (e.g., incomplete vs. complete burst fractures) when evaluating the outcomes of removing or retaining pedicle screw instruments after thoracolumbar burst fractures, which would help to observe actual clinical outcomes and avoid confusing the effects of fracture types. Additionally, pedicle screw removal is a second surgery performed under general anesthesia, which has substantial economic implications; therefore, a cost-effectiveness analysis should also be performed for policymakers, decision-makers, and other stakeholders [52,69,71].

4.6. Limitations

This study has several weaknesses. First, there was substantial clinical heterogeneity among the included studies, including the patient populations (e.g., symptomatic or asymptomatic), the morphology and classification of thoracolumbar burst fractures (e.g., incomplete or complete burst fractures), the severity of injury (e.g., the degree of injury to the discs, the integrity of the posterior ligamentous complex), the treatment strategies of thoracolumbar burst fractures, criteria for implant removal, follow-up duration, etc. These discrepancies reflect the lack of consensus on thoracolumbar burst fractures and compromise the quality of evidence. Second, this study was predetermined to include all kinds of studies, including case reports and case series, which may induce remarkable publication bias, since studies with positive results (e.g., unexpected complications) are more likely to be published in peer-reviewed journals [71]. Third, 25 of 35 included studies were from Asia, mainly from China, Japan, and South Korea, which may also induce bias.

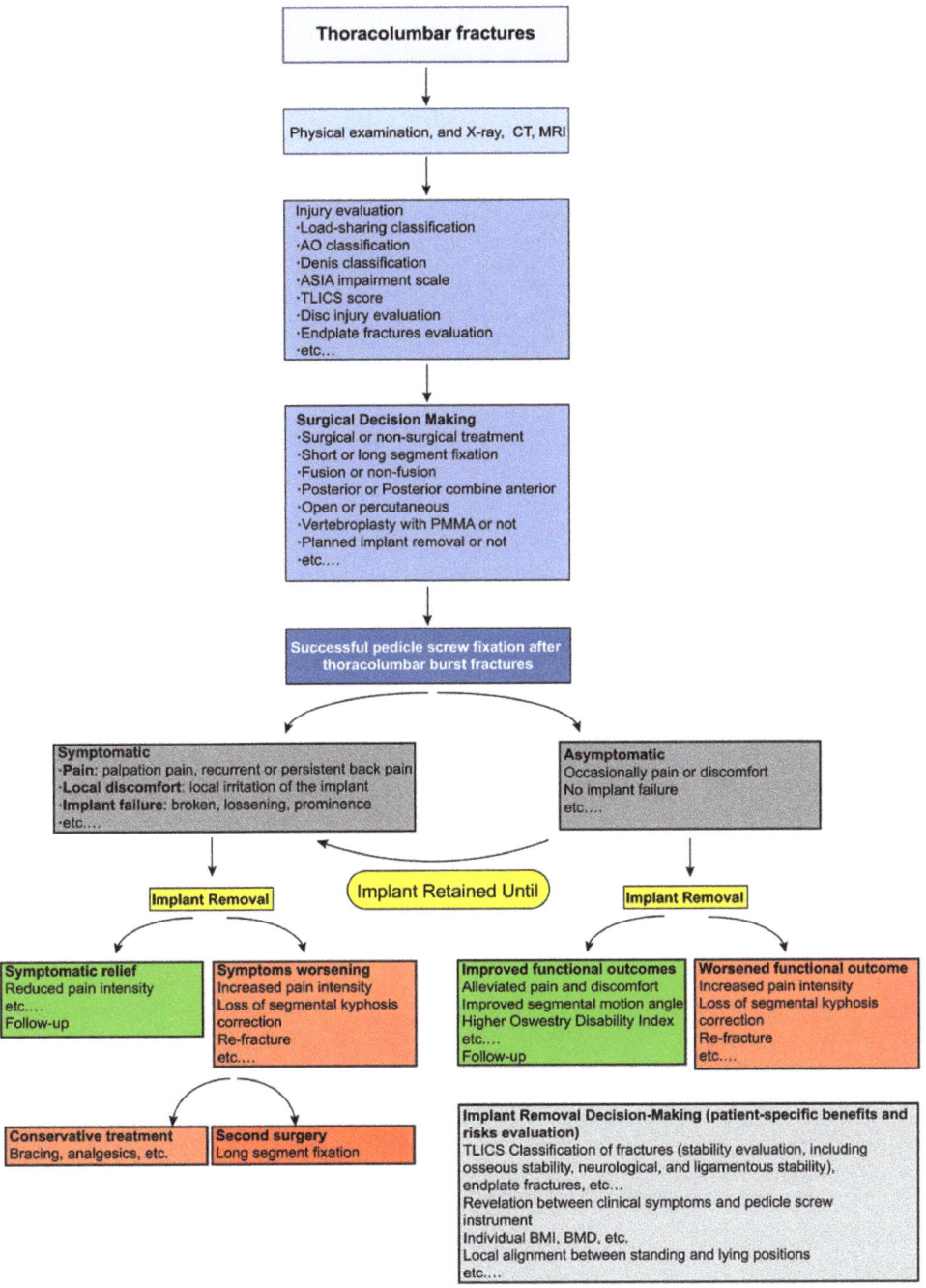

Figure 2. A proposed flow diagram for the management of thoracolumbar burst fractures. Abbreviations: CT, Computed Tomography; MRI, Magnetic Resonance Imaging; ASIA, American Spinal Injury Association; TLICS, Thoracolumbar Injury Classification and Severity; PMMA, Polymethyl Methacrylate; BMI, Body Mass Index; BMD, Bone Mineral Density.

5. Conclusions

In conclusion, the removal of implants after successful fusion of thoracolumbar burst fractures may be performed effectively to restore flexibility and relieve pain, but it may also lead to the progression of kyphotic deformity and surgical complications. Both surgeons and patients should be aware of the indications and have appropriate expectations of the benefits and risks of implant removal. There was no robust evidence to support the routine removal of pedicle screw instruments after the successful fusion of thoracolumbar burst fractures, which may expose the patients to unnecessary complications and costs. The potential benefits and possible risks should be weighed to support patient-specific clinical decision-making. Further research is warranted to provide more evidence to clarify this issue.

Supplementary Materials: The following supporting information can be downloaded at: https://www.mdpi.com/article/10.3390/jcm12062213/s1, Table S1: Search strategies for primary databases; Table S2: Baseline characteristics of the included case reports and case series; Table S3: The reported clinical outcomes in case reports and case series.

Author Contributions: X.W.: Contributed substantially to conception and design, acquisition of data, analysis, and interpretation of data; drafted the article; gave final approval of the version to be published; agreed to act as a guarantor of the work. X.-D.W.: Contributed substantially to conception and design, acquisition of data, analysis, and interpretation of data; drafted the article; gave final approval of the version to be published; agreed to act as a guarantor of the work. Y.Z.: Contributed substantially to the acquisition and interpretation of data; revised it critically for valuable intellectual content; gave final approval of the version to be published; agreed to act as a guarantor of the work. Z.Z.: Contributed substantially to the acquisition and interpretation of data; revised it critically for valuable intellectual content; gave final approval of the version to be published; agreed to act as a guarantor of the work. J.J.: Contributed substantially to the acquisition and interpretation of data; revised it critically for valuable intellectual content; gave final approval of the version to be published; agreed to act as a guarantor of the work. G.L.: Contributed substantially to the acquisition and interpretation of data; revised it critically for valuable intellectual content; gave final approval of the version to be published; agreed to act as a guarantor of the work. J.L.: Contributed substantially to the acquisition and interpretation of data; revised it critically for valuable intellectual content; gave final approval of the version to be published; agreed to act as a guarantor of the work. J.S.: Contributed substantially to the acquisition and interpretation of data; revised it critically for valuable intellectual content; gave final approval of the version to be published; agreed to act as a guarantor of the work. Y.S.: Contributed substantially to conception and design, acquisition of data, analysis, and interpretation of data; revised it critically for valuable intellectual content; gave final approval of the version to be published; agreed to act as a guarantor of the work. All authors have read and agreed to the published version of the manuscript.

Funding: This study was supported by the Beijing Jishuitan Hospital Natural Fund Incubation Program (Grant No. ZR-202304), Beijing Municipal Science & Technology Commission (Grant No. Z191100004419007), and Beijing Jishuitan Hospital Research Funding (Grant No. XKGG201811).

Institutional Review Board Statement: This was a systematic review, and no ethics approval and consent to participate were required.

Informed Consent Statement: Not applicable.

Data Availability Statement: The datasets used and analyzed during the study will be available from the corresponding authors on reasonable request.

Conflicts of Interest: The authors declare no conflict of interest.

Abbreviations

ASIA	American Spinal Injury Association
BMD	Bone Mineral Density
BMI	Body Mass Index
CIs	Confidence Intervals
CT	Computed Tomography
MD	Mean Difference
MeSH	Medical Subject Headings
MRI	Magnetic Resonance Imaging
NOS	Newcastle-Ottawa Scale
ODI	Oswestry Disability Index
PMMA	Polymethyl Methacrylate
PRISMA	Preferred Reporting Items for Systematic Reviews and Meta-Analyses
ROM	Range of Motion
RRs	Risk Ratios
SF-36	Short Form 36
SMD	Standardized Mean Difference
TLICS	Thoracolumbar Injury Classification and Severity
VAS	Visual Analogue Scale

References

1. Bouxsein, M.; Genant, H. *The Breaking Spine*; International Osteoporosis Foundation: Nyon, Switzerland, 2010.
2. Hu, R.; Mustard, C.A.; Burns, C. Epidemiology of incident spinal fracture in a complete population. *Spine* **1996**, *21*, 492–499. [CrossRef] [PubMed]
3. Dai, L.-Y.; Jiang, S.-D.; Wang, X.-Y.; Jiang, L.-S.A. Review of the management of thoracolumbar burst fractures. *Surg. Neurol.* **2007**, *67*, 221–231. [CrossRef] [PubMed]
4. Gnanenthiran, S.R.; Adie, S.; Harris, I.A. Nonoperative versus operative treatment for thoracolumbar burst fractures without neurologic deficit: A meta-analysis. *Clin. Orthop. Relat. Res.* **2012**, *470*, 567–577. [CrossRef]
5. Siebenga, J.; Leferink, V.J.; Segers, M.J.; Elzinga, M.J.; Bakker, F.C.; Henk, J.T.M.; Rommens, P.M.; ten Duis, H.-J.; Patka, P. Treatment of traumatic thoracolumbar spine fractures: A multicenter prospective randomized study of operative versus nonsurgical treatment. *Spine* **2006**, *31*, 2881–2890. [CrossRef]
6. Pehlivanoglu, T.; Akgul, T.; Bayram, S.; Meric, E.; Ozdemir, M.; Korkmaz, M.; Sar, C. Conservative Versus Operative Treatment of Stable Thoracolumbar Burst Fractures in Neurologically Intact Patients: Is There Any Difference Regarding the Clinical and Radiographic Outcomes? *Spine* **2020**, *45*, 452–458. [CrossRef] [PubMed]
7. Kumar, A.; Aujla, R.; Lee, C. The management of thoracolumbar burst fractures: A prospective study between conservative management, traditional open spinal surgery and minimally interventional spinal surgery. *Springerplus* **2015**, *4*, 204. [CrossRef]
8. Wood, K.; Bohn, D.; Mehbod, A. Anterior versus posterior treatment of stable thoracolumbar burst fractures without neurologic deficit: A prospective, randomized study. *Clin. Spine Surg.* **2005**, *18*, S15–S23. [CrossRef] [PubMed]
9. Hitchon, P.W.; Torner, J.; Eichholz, K.M.; Beeler, S.N. Comparison of anterolateral and posterior approaches in the management of thoracolumbar burst fractures. *J. Neurosurg. Spine* **2006**, *5*, 117–125. [CrossRef] [PubMed]
10. Sapkas, G.; Kateros, K.; Papadakis, S.A.; Brilakis, E.; Macheras, G.; Katonis, P. Treatment of unstable thoracolumbar burst fractures by indirect reduction and posterior stabilization: Short-segment versus long-segment stabilization. *Open Orthop. J.* **2010**, *4*, 7. [CrossRef]
11. Dai, L.-Y.; Jiang, L.-S.; Jiang, S.-D. Posterior short-segment fixation with or without fusion for thoracolumbar burst fractures: A five to seven-year prospective randomized study. *J. Bone Jt. Surg.* **2009**, *91*, 1033–1041. [CrossRef]
12. Tian, N.-F.; Wu, Y.-S.; Zhang, X.-L.; Wu, X.-L.; Chi, Y.-L.; Mao, F.-M. Fusion versus nonfusion for surgically treated thoracolumbar burst fractures: A meta-analysis. *PLoS ONE* **2013**, *8*, e63995. [CrossRef]
13. Denis, F. The three column spine and its significance in the classification of acute thoracolumbar spinal injuries. *Spine* **1983**, *8*, 817–831. [CrossRef]
14. Kim, B.-G.; Dan, J.-M.; Shin, D.-E. Treatment of thoracolumbar fracture. *Asian Spine J.* **2015**, *9*, 133. [CrossRef] [PubMed]
15. Cahueque, M.; Cobar, A.; Zuñiga, C.; Caldera, G. Management of burst fractures in the thoracolumbar spine. *J. Orthop.* **2016**, *13*, 278–281. [CrossRef] [PubMed]
16. Heary, R.F.; Kumar, S. Decision-making in burst fractures of the thoracolumbar and lumbar spine. *Indian J. Orthop.* **2007**, *41*, 268. [CrossRef] [PubMed]
17. Minkowitz, R.B.; Bhadsavle, S.; Walsh, M.; Egol, K.A. Removal of painful orthopaedic implants after fracture union. *J. Bone Jt. Surg.* **2007**, *89*, 1906–1912. [CrossRef]
18. Hanson, B.; van der Werken, C.; Stengel, D. Surgeons' beliefs and perceptions about removal of orthopaedic implants. *BMC Musculoskelet. Disord.* **2008**, *9*, 73. [CrossRef]

19. Wild, A.; Pinto, M.R.; Butler, L.; Bressan, C.; Wroblewski, J.M. Removal of lumbar instrumentation for the treatment of recurrent low back pain in the absence of pseudarthrosis. *Arch. Orthop. Trauma Surg.* **2003**, *123*, 414–418.
20. Gaine, W.J.; Andrew, S.M.; Chadwick, P.; Cooke, E.; Williamson, J.B. Late operative site pain with isola posterior instrumentation requiring implant removal: Infection or metal reaction? *Spine* **2001**, *26*, 583–587. [CrossRef]
21. Reith, G.; Schmitz-Greven, V.; Hensel, K.O.; Schneider, M.M.; Tinschmann, T.; Bouillon, B.; Probst, C. Metal implant removal: Benefits and drawbacks–a patient survey. *BMC Surg.* **2015**, *15*, 96. [CrossRef]
22. Hahn, F.; Zbinden, R.; Min, K. Late implant infections caused by Propionibacterium acnes in scoliosis surgery. *Eur. Spine J.* **2005**, *14*, 783–788. [CrossRef]
23. Jamil, W.; Allami, M.; Choudhury, M.; Mann, C.; Bagga, T.; Roberts, A. Do orthopaedic surgeons need a policy on the removal of metalwork? A descriptive national survey of practicing surgeons in the United Kingdom. *Injury* **2008**, *39*, 362–367. [CrossRef]
24. Bostman, O.; Pihlajamaki, H. Routine implant removal after fracture surgery: A potentially reducible consumer of hospital resources in trauma units. *J. Trauma* **1996**, *41*, 846–849. [CrossRef]
25. Niu, S.; Yang, D.; Ma, Y.; Lin, S.; Xu, X. Is removal of the internal fixation after successful intervertebral fusion necessary? A case-control study based on patient-reported quality of life. *J. Orthop. Surg. Res.* **2022**, *17*, 141. [CrossRef] [PubMed]
26. Tanasansomboon, T.; Kittipibul, T.; Limthongkul, W.; Yingsakmongkol, W.; Kotheeranurak, V.; Singhatanadgige, W. Thoracolumbar Burst Fracture without Neurological Deficit: Review of Controversies and Current Evidence of Treatment. *World Neurosurg.* **2022**, *162*, 29–35. [CrossRef] [PubMed]
27. Higgins, J.P.T.; Green, S. (Eds.) *Cochrane Handbook for Systematic Reviews of Interventions*, version 5.1.0 [updated March 2011]; John Wiley & Sons: Chichester, UK, 2011; Available online: http://www.cochrane.org/handbook (accessed on 8 March 2016).
28. Moher, D.; Liberati, A.; Tetzlaff, J.; Altman, D.G. PRISMA Group Preferred reporting items for systematic reviews and meta-analyses: The PRISMA statement. *Int. J. Surg.* **2010**, *8*, 336–341. [CrossRef] [PubMed]
29. Wells, G.A.; Shea, B.; O'Connell, D.; Peterson, J.; Welch, V.; Losos, M.; Tugwell, P. The Newcastle-Ottawa Scale (NOS) for Assessing the Quality of Nonrandomised Studies in Meta-Analyses. Available online: https://www.ohri.ca/programs/clinical_epidemiology/oxford.asp (accessed on 24 February 2023).
30. Vanichkachorn, J.S.; Vaccaro, A.R.; Cohen, M.J.; Cotler, J.M. Potential large vessel injury during thoracolumbar pedicle screw removal: A case report. *Spine* **1997**, *22*, 110–113. [CrossRef]
31. Waelchli, B.; Min, K.; Cathrein, P.; Boos, N. Vertebral body compression fracture after removal of pedicle screws: A report of two cases. *Eur. Spine J.* **2002**, *11*, 504–506. [CrossRef]
32. Cappuccio, M.; De Iure, F.; Amendola, L.; Martucci, A. Vertebral body compression fracture after percutaneous pedicle screw removal in a young man. *J. Orthop. Traumatol.* **2015**, *16*, 343–345. [CrossRef]
33. Takeda, K.; Aoki, Y.; Nakajima, T.; Sato, Y.; Sato, M.; Yoh, S.; Takahashi, H.; Nakajima, A.; Eguchi, Y.; Orita, S.; et al. Postoperative loss of correction after combined posterior and anterior spinal fusion surgeries in a lumbar burst fracture patient with Class II obesity. *Surg. Neurol. Int.* **2022**, *13*, 210. [CrossRef]
34. Kim, S.W.; Ju, C.I.; Kim, C.G.; Lee, S.M.; Shin, H. Efficacy of spinal implant removal after thoracolumbar junction fusion. *J. Korean Neurosurg. Soc.* **2008**, *43*, 139. [CrossRef] [PubMed]
35. Wang, X.-Y.; Dai, L.-Y.; Xu, H.-Z.; Chi, Y.-L. Kyphosis recurrence after posterior short-segment fixation in thoracolumbar burst fractures. *J. Neurosurg. Spine* **2008**, *8*, 246–254. [CrossRef]
36. Toyone, T.; Ozawa, T.; Inada, K.; Shirahata, T.; Shiboi, R.; Watanabe, A.; Matsuki, K.; Hasue, F.; Fujiyoshi, T.; Aoki, Y.; et al. Short-segment fixation without fusion for thoracolumbar burst fractures with neurological deficit can preserve thoracolumbar motion without resulting in post-traumatic disc degeneration: A 10-year follow-up study. *Spine* **2013**, *38*, 1482–1490. [CrossRef] [PubMed]
37. Axelsson, P.; Strömqvist, B. Can implant removal restore mobility after fracture of the thoracolumbar segment? A radiostereometric study. *Acta Orthop.* **2016**, *87*, 511–515. [CrossRef] [PubMed]
38. Knop, C.; Fabian, H.F.; Bastian, L.; Blauth, M. Late results of thoracolumbar fractures after posterior instrumentation and transpedicular bone grafting. *Spine* **2001**, *26*, 88–99. [CrossRef]
39. Song, K.-J.; Kim, K.-H.; Lee, S.-K.; Kim, J.-R. Clinical efficacy of implant removal after posterior spinal arthrodesis with pedicle screw fixation for the thoracolumbar burst fractures. *J. Korean Orthop. Assoc.* **2007**, *42*, 808–814. [CrossRef]
40. Xu, B.S.; Tang, T.S.; Yang, H.L. Long-term results of thoracolumbar and lumbar burst fractures after short-segment pedicle instrumentation, with special reference to implant failure and correction loss. *Orthop. Surg.* **2009**, *1*, 85–93. [CrossRef]
41. Stavridis, S.I.; Bücking, P.; Schaeren, S.; Jeanneret, B.; Schnake, K.J. Implant removal after posterior stabilization of the thoracolumbar spine. *Arch. Orthop. Trauma Surg.* **2010**, *130*, 119. [CrossRef]
42. Yang, H.; Shi, J.H.; Ebraheim, M.; Liu, X.; Konrad, J.; Husain, I.; Tang, T.S.; Liu, J. Outcome of thoracolumbar burst fractures treated with indirect reduction and fixation without fusion. *Eur. Spine J.* **2011**, *20*, 380–386. [CrossRef]
43. Wang, J.; Zhou, Y.; Zhang, Z.F.; Li, C.Q.; Zheng, W.J.; Liu, J. Radiological study on disc degeneration of thoracolumbar burst fractures treated by percutaneous pedicle screw fixation. *Eur. Spine J.* **2013**, *22*, 489–494. [CrossRef]
44. Kim, H.S.; Kim, S.W.; Ju, C.I.; Wang, H.S.; Lee, S.M.; Kim, D.M. Implant removal after percutaneous short segment fixation for thoracolumbar burst fracture: Does it preserve motion? *J. Korean Neurosurg. Soc.* **2014**, *55*, 73–77. [CrossRef]
45. Ko, S.-B.; Lee, S.-W. Result of posterior instrumentation without fusion in the management of thoracolumbar and lumbar unstable burst fracture. *Clin. Spine Surg.* **2014**, *27*, 189–195. [CrossRef] [PubMed]

46. Jeon, C.-H.; Lee, H.-D.; Lee, Y.-S.; Seo, J.-H.; Chung, N.-S. Is it beneficial to remove the pedicle screw instrument after successful posterior fusion of thoracolumbar burst fractures? *Spine* **2015**, *40*, E627–E633. [CrossRef]
47. Aono, H.; Tobimatsu, H.; Ariga, K.; Kuroda, M.; Nagamoto, Y.; Takenaka, S.; Furuya, M.; Iwasaki, M. Surgical outcomes of temporary short-segment instrumentation without augmentation for thoracolumbar burst fractures. *Injury* **2016**, *47*, 1337–1344. [CrossRef] [PubMed]
48. Chen, J.X.; Xu, D.L.; Sheng, S.R.; Goswami, A.; Xuan, J.; Jin, H.M.; Chen, J.; Chen, Y.; Zheng, Z.M.; Chen, X.B.; et al. Risk factors of kyphosis recurrence after implant removal in thoracolumbar burst fractures following posterior short-segment fixation. *Int. Orthop.* **2016**, *40*, 1253–1260. [CrossRef] [PubMed]
49. Chou, P.H.; Ma, H.L.; Liu, C.L.; Wang, S.T.; Lee, O.K.; Chang, M.C.; Yu, W.K. Is removal of the implants needed after fixation of burst fractures of the thoracolumbar and lumbar spine without fusion? a retrospective evaluation of radiological and functional outcomes. *Bone Jt. J.* **2016**, *98-B*, 109–116. [CrossRef]
50. Aono, H.; Ishii, K.; Tobimatsu, H.; Nagamoto, Y.; Takenaka, S.; Furuya, M.; Chiaki, H.; Iwasaki, M. Temporary short-segment pedicle screw fixation for thoracolumbar burst fractures: Comparative study with or without vertebroplasty. *Spine J.* **2017**, *17*, 1113–1119. [CrossRef]
51. Hoppe, S.; Aghayev, E.; Ahmad, S.; Keel, M.J.B.; Ecker, T.M.; Deml, M.; Benneker, L.M. Short Posterior Stabilization in Combination With Cement Augmentation for the Treatment of Thoracolumbar Fractures and the Effects of Implant Removal. *Glob. Spine J.* **2017**, *7*, 317–324. [CrossRef]
52. Lee, H.-D.; Jeon, C.-H.; Chung, N.-S.; Seo, Y.-W. Cost-utility analysis of pedicle screw removal after successful posterior instrumented fusion in thoracolumbar burst fractures. *Spine* **2017**, *42*, E926–E932. [CrossRef]
53. Smits, A.; Den Ouden, L.; Jonkergouw, A.; Deunk, J.; Bloemers, F. Posterior implant removal in patients with thoracolumbar spine fractures: Long-term results. *Eur. Spine J.* **2017**, *26*, 1525–1534. [CrossRef]
54. Aono, H.; Ishii, K.; Takenaka, S.; Tobimatsu, H.; Nagamoto, Y.; Horii, C.; Yamashita, T.; Furuya, M.; Iwasaki, M. Risk factors for a kyphosis recurrence after short-segment temporary posterior fixation for thoracolumbar burst fractures. *J. Clin. Neurosci.* **2019**, *66*, 138–143. [CrossRef] [PubMed]
55. Oh, H.S.; Seo, H.Y. Percutaneous Pedicle Screw Fixation in Thoracolumbar Fractures: Comparison of Results According to Implant Removal Time. *Clin. Orthop. Surg.* **2019**, *11*, 291–296. [CrossRef]
56. Chen, L.; Liu, H.; Hong, Y.; Yang, Y.; Hu, L. Minimally Invasive Decompression and Intracorporeal Bone Grafting Combined with Temporary Percutaneous Short-Segment Pedicle Screw Fixation for Treatment of Thoracolumbar Burst Fracture with Neurological Deficits. *World Neurosurg.* **2020**, *135*, e209–e220. [CrossRef]
57. Hou, G.J.; Zhou, F.; Tian, Y.; Ji, H.Q.; Zhang, Z.S.; Guo, Y.; Lv, Y.; Yang, Z.W.; Zhang, Y.W. Risk factors of recurrent kyphosis in thoracolumbar burst fracture patients treated by short segmental pedicle screw fixation. *Beijing Da Xue Xue Bao Yi Xue Ban* **2020**, *53*, 167–174.
58. Ko, S.; Jung, S.; Song, S.; Kim, J.Y.; Kwon, J. Long-term follow-up results in patients with thoracolumbar unstable burst fracture treated with temporary posterior instrumentation without fusion and implant removal surgery: Follow-up results for at least 10 years. *Medicine* **2020**, *99*, e19780. [CrossRef] [PubMed]
59. Manson, N.; El-Mughayyar, D.; Bigney, E.; Richardson, E.; Abraham, E. Instrumentation Removal following Minimally Invasive Posterior Percutaneous Pedicle Screw-Rod Stabilization (PercStab) of Thoracolumbar Fractures Is Not Always Required. *Adv. Orthop.* **2020**, *2020*, 7949216. [CrossRef] [PubMed]
60. Sasagawa, T.; Takagi, Y.; Hayashi, H.; Nanpo, K. Patient Satisfaction with Implant Removal after Stabilization Using Percutaneous Pedicle Screws for Traumatic Thoracolumbar Fracture. *Asian J. Neurosurg.* **2021**, *16*, 765–769. [CrossRef] [PubMed]
61. Hirahata, M.; Kitagawa, T.; Yasui, Y.; Oka, H.; Yamamoto, I.; Yamada, K.; Fujita, M.; Kawano, H.; Ishii, K. Vacuum phenomenon as a predictor of kyphosis after implant removal following posterior pedicle screw fixation without fusion for thoracolumbar burst fracture: A single-center retrospective study. *BMC Musculoskelet. Disord.* **2022**, *23*, 94. [CrossRef]
62. Kenfack, Y.; Oduguwa, E.; Barrie, U.; Kafka, B.; Tecle, N.; Neely, O.; Bagley, C.; Aoun, S. P173: Implications, benefits, and risks of hardware removal following percutaneous screw fixation for thoracolumbar fractures: A retrospective case series of 58 patients at a single institution. *Glob. Spine J.* **2022**, *12* (Suppl. S294), 3.
63. Wu, J.; Zhu, J.; Wang, Z.; Jin, H.; Wang, Y.; Liu, B.; Yin, X.; Du, L.; Wang, Y.; Liu, M.; et al. Outcomes in Thoracolumbar and Lumbar Traumatic Fractures: Does Restoration of Unfused Segmental Mobility Correlated to Implant Removal Time? *World Neurosurg.* **2022**, *157*, e254–e263. [CrossRef]
64. Xu, X.; Cao, Y.; Fan, J.; Lv, Y.; Zhou, F.; Tian, Y.; Ji, H.; Zhang, Z.; Guo, Y.; Yang, Z.; et al. Is It Necessary to Remove the Implants After Fixation of Thoracolumbar and Lumbar Burst Fractures Without Fusion? A Retrospective Cohort Study of Elderly Patients. *Front. Surg.* **2022**, *9*, 921678. [CrossRef]
65. Kweh, B.T.S.; Tan, T.; Lee, H.Q.; Hunn, M.; Liew, S.; Tee, J.W. Implant Removal Versus Implant Retention Following Posterior Surgical Stabilization of Thoracolumbar Burst Fractures: A Systematic Review and Meta-Analysis. *Glob. Spine J.* **2022**, *12*, 700–718. [CrossRef] [PubMed]
66. Li, Y.; Shen, Z.; Huang, M.; Wang, X. Stepwise resection of the posterior ligamentous complex for stability of a thoracolumbar compression fracture: An in vitro biomechanical investigation. *Medicine* **2017**, *96*, e7873. [CrossRef] [PubMed]
67. Deckey, J.E.; Bradford, D.S. Loss of sagittal plane correction after removal of spinal implants. *Spine* **2000**, *25*, 2453–2460. [CrossRef] [PubMed]

68. Busam, M.L.; Esther, R.J.; Obremskey, W.T. Hardware removal: Indications and expectations. *J. Am. Acad. Orthop. Surg.* **2006**, *14*, 113–120. [CrossRef]
69. Vos, D.; Verhofstad, M. Indications for implant removal after fracture healing: A review of the literature. *Eur. J. Trauma Emerg. Surg.* **2013**, *39*, 327–337. [CrossRef]
70. Kim, G.W.; Jang, J.W.; Hur, H.; Lee, J.K.; Kim, J.H.; Kim, S.H. Predictive factors for a kyphosis recurrence following short-segment pedicle screw fixation including fractured vertebral body in unstable thoracolumbar burst fractures. *J. Korean Neurosurg. Soc.* **2014**, *56*, 230–236. [CrossRef]
71. Mahid, S.S.; Qadan, M.; Hornung, C.A.; Galandiuk, S. Assessment of publication bias for the surgeon scientist. *Br. J. Surg.* **2008**, *95*, 943–949. [CrossRef]

Disclaimer/Publisher's Note: The statements, opinions and data contained in all publications are solely those of the individual author(s) and contributor(s) and not of MDPI and/or the editor(s). MDPI and/or the editor(s) disclaim responsibility for any injury to people or property resulting from any ideas, methods, instructions or products referred to in the content.

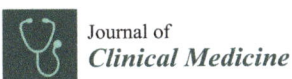

Viewpoint

Complete Intra-Operative Image Data Including 3D X-rays: A New Format for Surgical Papers Needed?

Pietro Regazzoni [1,*,†], Wen-Chih Liu [2,3], Jesse B. Jupiter [3,†] and Alberto A. Fernandez dell'Oca [4,5]

1. Department of Trauma Surgery, University Hospital Basel, 4031 Basel, Switzerland
2. Kaohsiung Medical University Hospital, Collage of Medicine, Kaohsiung Medical University, Kaohsiung 80756, Taiwan
3. Hand and Arm Center, Department of Orthopedics, Massachusetts General Hospital, Boston, MA 02114, USA
4. Department of Traumatology, British Hospital, Montevideo 11600, Uruguay
5. Residency Program in Traumatology and Orthopedics, University of Montevideo, Montevideo 11600, Uruguay
* Correspondence: p_regazzoni@bluewin.ch; Tel.: +41-(79)-6400286
† Pietro Regazzoni and Jesse B. Jupiter are professors emeriti.

Abstract: Intra-operative 3D X-rays have been confirmed to decrease revision rates and improve optimal screw placement in complex fractures of the distal radius. Compared with traditional surgical publications, another advantage of whole intraoperative clinical imaging can be presented in electronic databases, e.g., the ICUC working group, through a link without size limitation. The detail of complete intra-operative image dataset includes essential technical details which can be analyzed secondarily for costs and complications, considering the technical performance bias. Furthermore, the new format complies with reading/learning preferences of young surgeons and allows secondary work-up by artificial intelligence. Intra-operative 3D X-ray is a new approach for better surgical outcomes, economic benefit, and educational purposes.

Keywords: intra-operative 3D X-ray; intra-operative 3D CT; artificial intelligence; evidence-based surgery; distal radius fracture

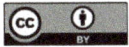

A publication by Halvachizadeh et al. [1] has confirmed the advantage of using intra-operative 3D imaging for complex fractures of the distal radius by enabling a decrease in revision rates and improved optimal screw placement without increasing duration of surgery. Previous papers have also shown the economic advantages of intra-operative 3D X-rays [2,3]. A further advantage—for learning—would result from allowing access not only to complete radiological but also clinical imaging, as proposed by the ICUC working group (www.icuc.net) [4]. Electronic publishing easily allows the management of the great amount of data resulting from the implementation of such a concept. Access to complete data would also positively influence quality control efforts by allowing the confrontation of results obtained from different sources under repeated, comparable conditions [5].

In conventional surgical publications—even following very precisely formulated research protocols for the highest evidence standard like RCT—essential data, e.g., reduction maneuvers in fracture treatment, are not accessible to the readers. Skills aspects are essential for the outcome, can be measured and correlated with complications and costs [6], but cannot be analyzed secondarily without complete intra-operative image data. The inter-operator variance in technical performance is a proven reality and inevitably produces a "technical performance bias" [7]. In simple procedure, a 3D X-ray may not be necessarily needed; however, the bias is particularly important for complex surgical procedures. This seems to be a fundamental problem of surgical trials and a fundamental obstacle to sound "evidence-based surgery". Efforts should be made to produce evidence levels similar to those well documented in clinical trials for new drug development.

Size limitations have hitherto led to the avoidance of complete intra-operative image documentations being shown in conventional surgical papers. Electronic formats have changed the situation. A short main text can show representative images, whereas the total data set can then be made accessible through a link. Such a new format also complies with reading/learning preferences of young surgeons and allows secondary work-up by artificial intelligence (AI) in highly efficient neuromorphic learning system [8,9]. Complete intra-operative image data, as proposed and realized by the ICUC working group [10,11], also allows the inclusion of essential technical details once novel surgical techniques are introduced to general public, i.e., when "non-early users" produce "real-world data". It is well known that certain complications appear in a second use phase, often due to small deviations from the technique presented and used by inventors and early users, when the public starts to use the new method.

In conclusion, 3D intra-operative imaging is a beneficial addition rather than a requirement. To reach evidence levels comparable to drug development process, surgical trials need to adopt documentation methods including also clinical, intra-operative images. Secondary analysis of such data allows the measurement of surgical skills, avoidance of technical performance biases, and improve homogeneity of trial groups. New electronic, open-source formats allow access to the complete dataset by links, avoiding the size limitations of conventional publication formats, but managing quality control and allowing post-publication data mining.

Author Contributions: Conceptualization, P.R.; writing—original draft preparation, P.R.; writing—review and editing, W.-C.L., J.B.J. and A.A.F.d. All authors have read and agreed to the published version of the manuscript.

Funding: This research received no external funding.

Institutional Review Board Statement: Not applicable.

Informed Consent Statement: Not applicable.

Data Availability Statement: The complete intra-operative image data mentioned in this study are openly available at https://www.icuc.net.

Conflicts of Interest: Pietro Regazzoni and Alberto A. Fernandez dell'Oca co-founded ICUC and Jesse B. Jupiter is the head of upper limb of ICUC.

References

1. Halvachizadeh, S.; Berk, T.; Pieringer, A.; Ried, E.; Hess, F.; Pfeifer, R.; Pape, H.-C.; Allemann, F. Is the Additional Effort for an Intraoperative CT Scan Justified for Distal Radius Fracture Fixations? A Comparative Clinical Feasibility Study. *J. Clin. Med.* **2020**, *9*, 2254. [CrossRef] [PubMed]
2. Atesok, K.; Finkelstein, J.; Khoury, A.; Peyser, A.; Weil, Y.; Liebergall, M.; Mosheiff, R. The use of intraoperative three-dimensional imaging (ISO-C-3D) in fixation of intraarticular fractures. *Injury* **2007**, *38*, 1163–1169. [CrossRef] [PubMed]
3. Bischoff, M.; Hebecker, A.; Hartwig, E.; Gebhard, F. Cost effectiveness of intraoperative three-dimensional imaging with a mobile surgical C-arm. *Unfallchirurg* **2004**, *107*, 712–715. [CrossRef] [PubMed]
4. Perren, S.M.; Regazzoni, P.; Fernandez, A.A. Biomechanical and biological aspects of defect treatment in fractures using helical plates. *Acta Chir. Orthop. Traumatol. Cechoslov.* **2014**, *81*, 267–271.
5. Rallison, S. What are Journals for? *Ann. R. Coll. Surg. Engl.* **2015**, *97*, 89–91. [CrossRef] [PubMed]
6. Birkmeyer, J.D.; Finks, J.F.; O'Reilly, A.; Oerline, M.; Carlin, A.M.; Nunn, A.R.; Dimick, J.; Banerjee, M.; Birkmeyer, N.J.; Michigan Bariatric Surgery, C. Surgical skill and complication rates after bariatric surgery. *N. Engl. J. Med.* **2013**, *369*, 1434–1442. [CrossRef] [PubMed]
7. Stulberg, J.J.; Huang, R.; Kreutzer, L.; Ban, K.; Champagne, B.J.; Steele, S.R.; Johnson, J.K.; Holl, J.L.; Greenberg, C.C.; Bilimoria, K.Y. Association Between Surgeon Technical Skills and Patient Outcomes. *JAMA Surg.* **2020**, *155*, 960–968. [CrossRef] [PubMed]
8. Kassem, H.; Alapatt, D.; Mascagni, P.; Karargyris, A.; Padoy, N. Federated Cycling (FedCy): Semi-supervised Federated Learning of Surgical Phases. *IEEE Trans. Med. Imaging* **2022**. [CrossRef] [PubMed]
9. Liu, T.Y.; Mahjoubfar, A.; Prusinski, D.; Stevens, L. Neuromorphic computing for content-based image retrieval. *PLoS ONE* **2022**, *17*, e0264364. [CrossRef] [PubMed]

10. Regazzoni, P.; Fernandez, A.; Perren, S.M. Assessment of intra-operative surgical performance: Proof of concept of complete intra-operative image documentation in orthopaedic trauma. *Injury* **2021**, *52*, 7–8. [CrossRef]
11. Regazzoni, P.; Perren, S.M.; Fernández, A. MIO Helical Plate: Technically Easy, Improving Biology and Mechanics of "Double Plating". 2018. Available online: https://www.icuc.net/static/media/41.4861a219.pdf (accessed on 23 October 2022).

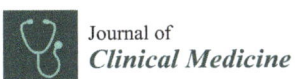

Case Report

Reconstruction of Chronic Proximal Hamstring Tear: A Novel Surgical Technique with Semitendinosus Tendon Allograft Assisted with Autologous Plasma Rich in Growth Factors (PRGF)

Antonio Ríos Luna [1,*], Homid Fahandezh-Saddi Díaz [2], Manuel Villanueva Martínez [3], Ángel Bueno Horcajadas [4], Roberto Prado [5], Eduardo Anitua [5] and Sabino Padilla [5]

1. Department of Traumatology and Orthopedic Surgery, Clínica Orthoindal, 04004 Almería, Spain
2. Department of Orthopedic Surgery, Hospital Universitario Fundación Alcorcón, 28922 Alcorcón, Spain
3. Department of Traumatology and Orthopedic Surgery, Avanfi Institute, 28015 Madrid, Spain
4. Department of Radiology, Hospital Universitario Fundación Alcorcón, 28922 Alcorcón, Spain
5. BTI—Biotechnology Institute I MAS D, 01007 Vitoria, Spain
* Correspondence: antoniorioslusna@gmail.com

Abstract: The reconstruction of a chronic proximal hamstring tear is a challenging pathology that posits difficulties to surgeons due to the distal retraction of the hamstring tendon stumps and the entrapment of the sciatic nerve within the scar formed around the torn hamstring tendon. We describe a novel surgical technique using a semitendinosus tendon allograft sutured in a "V inversion" manner, thereby avoiding an excess of tension and length of the new reconstructed hamstring tendons. In addition, and in order to speed up the healing process and avoid new sciatic entrapment, we assisted the surgery with liquid plasma rich in growth factors (PRGF) injected intraosseously, intratendinously and within the suture areas, as well as wrapping the sciatic nerve with a PRGF membrane. In conclusion, this novel approach offers mechanical and biological advantages to tackle the large retraction of hamstring stumps and the entrapment of the sciatic nerve within the scar.

Keywords: proximal hamstring avulsion; allograft reconstruction; chronic; PRGF; platelet-rich plasma; PRP

1. Introduction

A chronic proximal hamstring tear is a debilitating muscle injury associated with persistent pain, cramping, functional limitation, and weakness in the ischial (buttock) region, with more than 4–6 weeks of evolution [1]. The delayed diagnosis and the failed conservative treatments often result in a hamstring syndrome caused by the entrapment of the sciatic nerve within the scar formed around the torn hamstring tendon, causing an unrelenting pain that is exacerbated by prolonged sitting [2,3]. Moreover, the distal retraction of the hamstring tendon stumps of several centimeters makes the reinsertion of the entire conjoined tendon (JT) (made up of the long head of biceps femoris (LBF) and semitendinosus tendons (STT)) and the tendon of semimembranous muscle (SMT) extremely difficult [1,2].

In this manuscript, we describe a novel technique using a semitendinosus tendon allograft sutured in a "V inversion" manner, thereby avoiding an excess of tension and length of the new reconstructed hamstring tendons, which could lead to rupture at the suture areas. Moreover, and in order to enhance the repair process and avoid new sciatic entrapment, we assist the surgery with liquid plasma rich in growth factors (PRGF-Endoret) injected intraosseously, intratendinously, and within the suture areas, as well as wrapping the sciatic nerve with a PRGF membrane [4,5].

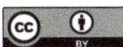

2. Case Report and Description of the Technique

2.1. Patient Presentation and Examination

A 45-year-old female with no medical history relevant to this injury underwent a motorcycle fall at low speed with the left lower extremity in hyperextension. She heard a snap, together with an acute intense cramping pain from the buttock region to the knee. Once at the hospital, the X-ray study did not show a bone fracture. She began a physiotherapy treatment, but, after a few days, the patient noticed a significant hematoma associated with a persistent pain (Figure 1a).

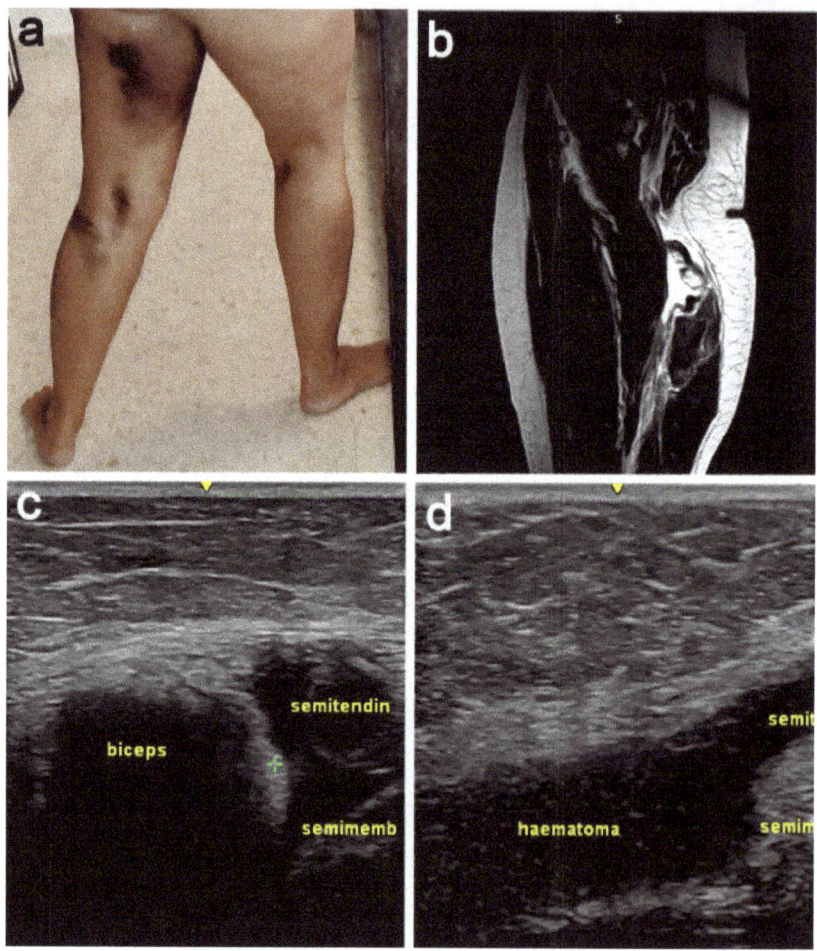

Figure 1. Preoperative description of the case. (**a**) Image of the haematoma two days after the accident, accompanied by lancinating pain with paresthesia similar to radicular pain. (**b**) MRI confirming the injury; the conjoint tendon was retracted 7 cm and the semimembranosus tendon 10 cm, with a significant accumulation of free fluid. (**c,d**) Ultrasound also showed complete disinsertion of both tendons, as well as their retraction.

In this second visit to the hospital, the performed US and MRI studies confirmed a complete detachment of conjoined tendon of biceps femoris and semitendinosus (JT), and the semimembranous tendon (SMT). After following a conservative treatment and 6 months after the accident, the patient came for the first time to our consultation reporting a significant functional limitation. Physical examination showed a limitation in knee extension while walking, a gap distal to the left gluteal fold, and the impossibility of knee flexion against resistance with a positive Puranen–Orava test. New MRI (Figure 1b) and US (Figure 1c,d) studies showed that the JT was retracted 7 cm and the SMT 10 cm. This injury could be classified as type 5-B following the classification developed by Wood et al. [6], namely, a complete tendon avulsion from bone with a retraction of the tendon ends associated with sciatic nerve involvement.

After discussing treatment options and possible outcomes, the patient underwent a surgical intervention with a novel technique using a semitendinosus tendon allograft in a "V inversion" manner assisted with liquid PRGF injected intraosseous, intratendinously and within the suture areas, and a PRGF membrane that wrapped the sciatic nerve.

2.2. Patient Positioning

After the induction of general anesthesia, the surgery was performed with the patient in the prone position, with the hip and knee at 20 and 30 degrees of flexion, respectively (Figure 2a). Previously, and in order to center the incision, we identified the stumps of the conjoined tendon (Biceps and semitendinosus) and SMT stumps with the aid of US and MRI (Figure 2b). In our patient, the distance between the ischial tuberosity and the gluteus fold was 3 cm, whereas the joint tendon and SMT were 7 and 10 cm away from the ischial tuberosity, respectively. Once the sterile prepping and draping were completed, the entire extremity was draped so that we could manipulate the hip and knee joints during the surgery to assess and adjust the graft tensioning.

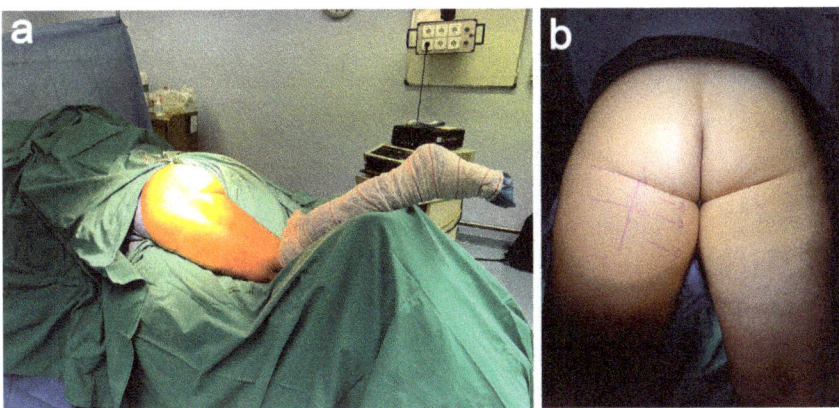

Figure 2. (a) The patient is placed in prone position with the hip and knee flexed. (b) Previously, the relevant anatomical structures are located.

2.3. Dissection, Neurolysis, and Tenolysis

A longitudinal/vertical incision was performed guided by the landmarks obtained with the aid of US and MRI. After dissecting the subcutaneous tissues, we identified the ischial tuberosity, torn hamstring tendons, and the entrapped sciatic nerve (Figure 3a). We carried out a careful distal-to-proximal exoneurolysis of the sciatic nerve and placed vessel-loops to visualize and avoid iatrogenic injury to the nerve during the surgery. Once identifying the stumps of both tendons that were retracted and entrapped by fibrotic tissue, we performed a careful tenolysis to free up both tendon stumps and freshen both stumps. In addition, we put Vicryl (Ethicon, Somerville, NJ, USA) sutures in each tendon stump, which served as control of the torn hamstring (Figure 3b).

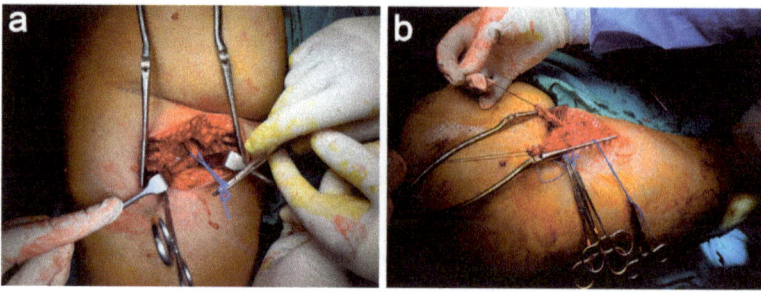

Figure 3. Dissection, neurolysis, and tenolysis (**a**) After exoneurolysis, the sciatic nerve is identified and placed laterally in the surgical field. (**b**) Following tenolysis, Vycril sutures are placed for traction on both tendons.

2.4. STT Allograft Preparation

Due to the impossibility of reinserting the hamstring tendon stumps into the ischial tuberosity, a free graft reconstruction with a 17 cm long STT allograft augmentation was carried out, allowing us to bridge the long gap (Figure 4a). The entire STT allograft was reinforced with a Hi-Fi Ribbon suture (ConMed, Largo, FL, USA), thereby endowing the reconstructed tendon augmentation with additional strength. The STT allograft was bent on itself, generating a double-thickness tendon allograft whose proximal section of 3 cm was reinforced with 2/0 Ethibond sutures (Ethicon, Somerville, NJ, USA), from which, were the two branches of the allograft stem toward the distal hamstring stumps in a "V inversion" shape (Figure 4b).

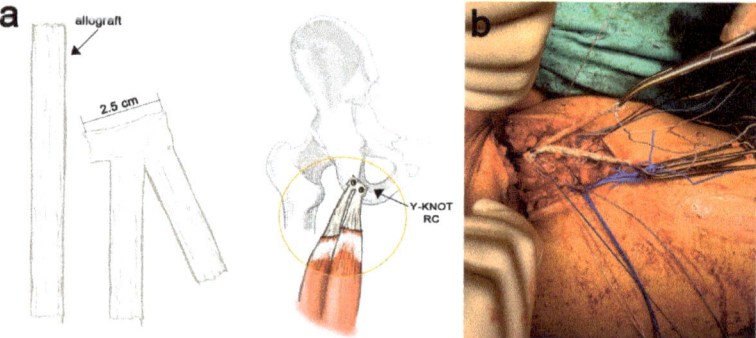

Figure 4. Semitendinosus tendon allograft preparation. (**a**) Description of allograft preparation and placement. (**b**) Intraoperative image showing the two branches of the allograft (inverted V-shaped).

2.5. STT Allograft Placement

After identification, dissection, and protection of the sciatic nerve, and following the correct anatomically location, we prepared the bony surface of the ischial tuberosity by curettage and rasp. Then, two self-punching Y-Knot RC (ConMed, Largo, FL, USA) suture anchors (two Hi-Fi, one blue and one white) were placed in the ischial tuberosity (Figure 5a). The first Y-Knot RC anchor was placed in a lateral and anterior position (corresponding to the SMT that is lateral and 3.1 cm proximal-to-distal and 1.1 cm medial-to-lateral). The second Y-Knot RC anchor was placed in a more posterior and medial location (the JT is medial 2.7 cm proximal-to-distal and 1.8 cm medial-to-lateral).

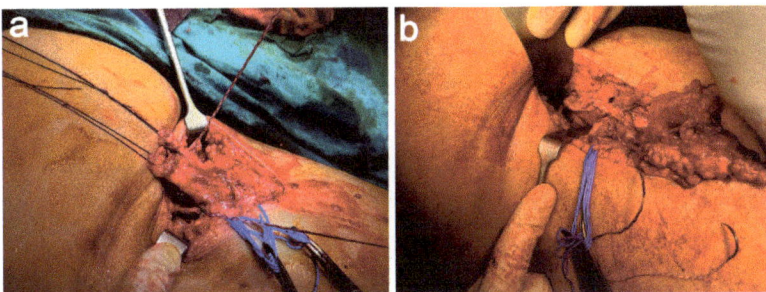

Figure 5. Semitendinosus tendon allograft placement. (**a**) Support with Ribbon resistance band. (**b**) Allograft to tendon suture.

Krakow type stitches were passed with the blue strand of a Y-Knot RC in the external arm of the "V" of the double reinforcement of the allograft. We performed the same but using the white strand at the base of the medial arm of the "V". As it is a sliding thread, by pulling on another thread of the same color that remains free, the graft slides and is placed in the anatomical position at the level of the ischial tuberosity. Once this double suture is secured, we made a medial and lateral reinforcement suture with the blue and white threads left over in each Y-Knot RC to provide significant solidity in the insertional area.

We then took the two tendon ends: the joint tendon on one side and the semimembranosus tendon on the other side. Next, we passed one of the distal ends of the allograft through the semimembranosus tendon (deeper) with a Pulvertaft-type suture. We checked the tension after the two passes, and we carefully mobilized the knee in a range of 60 degrees, which allowed us to assess the right tension of our suture. After verifying that it was satisfactory, we made two more passes to provide a strong suture. We repeated the procedure with the joint tendon and performed four tendon passes with the Pulvertaft-type technique (Figure 5b).

2.6. PRGF Preparation and Application

Platelet-rich plasma (PRP) was prepared according to the PRGF-Endoret method. PRGF is a leukocyte- and erythrocyte-free PRP with moderate platelet-enrichment [7]. Briefly, 72 mL of peripheral venous blood was withdrawn into 9 mL tubes containing 3.8% (wt/vol) sodium citrate (Endoret Traumatology kit, BTI Biotechnology Institute, Vitoria, Spain) before starting the patient's anesthesia. Then, the blood was centrifuged for 8 min at 580 g at room temperature in a System V centrifuge (BTI Biotechnology Institute, Vitoria, Spain). After centrifugation, three layers were obtained (plasma, buffy coat and packed red blood cells). The upper layer of plasma (F1 fraction) was collected in order to prepare the PRGF membrane. The 2 mL plasma fraction located just above the buffy coat (F2 fraction) was collected, avoiding the leukocyte layer, and was used to perform infiltrations.

We performed intraosseous (4 mL into the ischial tuberosity once freshened) and intratendinous infiltrations (8 mL) of liquid PRGF into the suture-repair areas (Figure 6a) The F2 fraction was activated in a time-controlled way by the addition of PRGF activator (10% $CaCl_2$) just before to these infiltrations performed with a 21 G $-$ 0.8 $\times$ 40 mm needle. Finally, the sciatic nerve was wrapped with a PRGF membrane (Figure 6b) elaborated with 8 mL of liquid F1, which was activated with 160 µL of PRGF activator and maintained for at least 15 min at room temperature until the formation of a clot.

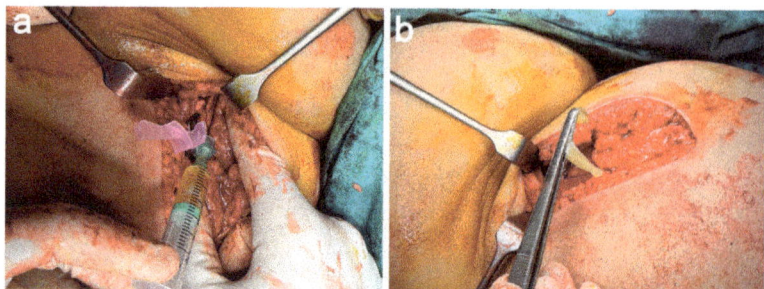

Figure 6. Application of PRGF. (**a**) Intratendinous infiltration of PRGF into the allograft suture-repair areas. (**b**) The sciatic nerve is wrapped with a PRGF membrane.

Furthermore, seven and fourteen days after the surgery, and assisted by US, we performed two infiltrations of PRGF in the sutured areas of the graft. In both cases, 8 mL of freshly activated F2 PRGF was infiltrated [4,5].

2.7. Postoperative Rehabilitation

The patient was kept in a hip and knee brace locked at 70 degrees and 30 degrees of flexion, respectively, for 8 weeks, not allowing the weight-bearing walk and using two crutches (Figure 7a). After 8 weeks, we removed the hip and knee brace and the patient underwent a rehabilitation program with a passive progressive range of motion of the hip and knee, allowing partial weight-bearing using two crutches. The US performed at week 12 showed images compatible with the integration of the allograft into the tendon (Figure 7b), which was the start point of an active rehabilitation program (Figure 7c). In a gradual manner, and always supervised by the physiotherapist and surgeon advice, our patient initiated quadriceps and hamstring isometric, eccentric and proprioceptive exercises, as well as active resistance strength exercises. After 12 months, the patient resumed her active lifestyle without any limitation.

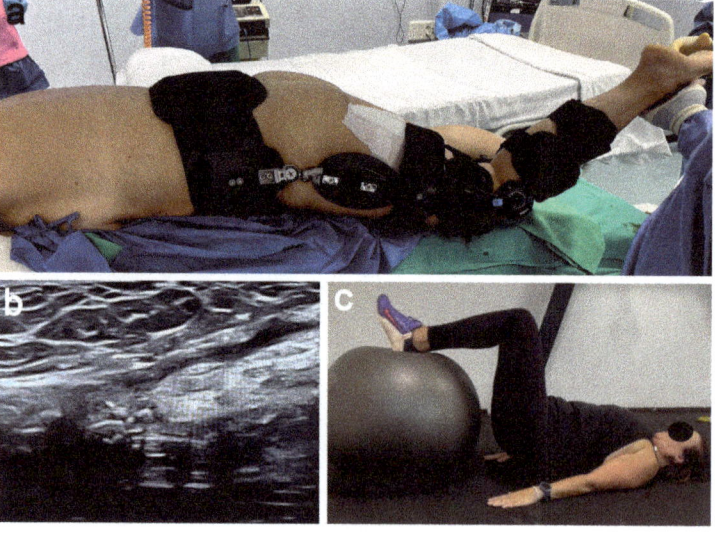

Figure 7. Postoperative rehabilitation. (**a**) Immobilizing splints keeping the knee and hip flexed. (**b**) US (week 12 postoperatively) showed images compatible with the integration of the allograft. (**c**) Rehabilitation process starting at 12 weeks.

3. Discussion

We describe the reconstruction of a chronic proximal hamstring tear using a semitendinosus tendon allograft sutured in a "V inversion" manner and assisted with PRGF as a novel surgical technique to treat a chronic proximal hamstring tear. Our patient resumed her active lifestyle without any limitation 12 months after the surgery. This new technique offers mechanical and biological advantages to tackle the large retraction of hamstring stumps and the entrapment of the sciatic nerve within the scar. In fact, 9 months after the surgery, the patient resumed her previous lifestyle, including recreational sport.

There have been reported numerous different procedures to overcome and bridge tear gaps superior to 5 cm between the tendon stumps and the ischial tuberosity in chronic proximal hamstring tears by using ipsilateral distal hamstring autografts [8] or Achilles tendon allografts [9], both with good post-operative clinical outcomes and patient satisfaction with 24 and 48-month (long term) follow-ups. Despite some inherent potential drawback of allografts, including infection and disease transmission, issues with the osseointegration and the cost and shortage of allografts, the surgical repair of retracted stumps superior to 5 cm is recommended and often necessary [2,9]. We chose to use a semitendinosus tendon allograft of 17 cm due to the dimensions of the stump retractions of 7 and 10 cm. In doing so, it endowed the reconstructed tendon augmentation with a controlled suture tension and the correct anatomically location at the proximal insertion, thereby recreating the native insertion at the ischial tuberosity [2]. Significantly, the Y-Knot RC anchor associated with robust sutures allow loads superior to 200 N, and having this type of fixation emerged as the gold standard treatment [10]. Moreover, the longitudinal/vertical incision guided by the landmarks obtained with the aid of US and MRI gave us enough room to perform the surgery accurately, assessing the tension of the suture anchors and the sutured stumps, as well as the use of PRGF in different surgical steps. The PRGF supplied the suture anchor and sutured stumps with trophic molecules that have been reported to promote the osseointegration of the graft, a better remodeling and the secretion of extracellular matrix, while avoiding fibrosis at the suture stumps as well as around the sciatic nerve, all effects leading to enhance the repair process [4,11–13]. At this point, and following Sanchez et al. [14], one improvement to add would be to soak in and infiltrate the allograft into the PRGF supernatant. However, this novel technique is not exempt from some pitfalls, mainly stemming from the long vertical incision and the period of 8 weeks wearing the hip and knee brace, the latter being cumbersome and hard to tolerate for patients. We consider that it is not recommended to shorten this time, as the immobilization time depends on the type of tendon sutured, the type of suture and whether or not allografting is required. In our case, these are very powerful tendons that require and demand a lot of strength, and the time described should be respected to avoid the risk of dehiscence or suture failure. A long longitudinal incision is recommended in chronic proximal hamstring tears when the tear distal gap of the hamstring tendon stumps assessed by US and MRI is several centimeters [2].

4. Conclusions

The PRGF-assisted reconstruction of chronic proximal hamstring tears with a semitendinosus tendon allograft provides mechanical and biological advantages to tackle the large retraction of hamstring stumps and the entrapment of the sciatic nerve within the scar.

Author Contributions: Conceptualization, A.R.L.; methodology, A.R.L., H.F.-S.D., M.V.M., Á.B.H., R.P., E.A. and S.P.; writing—original draft, S.P. and R.P.; writing—review and editing, A.R.L., H.F.-S.D., M.V.M., Á.B.H., R.P., E.A. and S.P. All authors have read and agreed to the published version of the manuscript.

Funding: This research received no external funding.

Institutional Review Board Statement: For this type of study (case report), formal ethical approval is not required.

Informed Consent Statement: The authors obtained the written consent of the patient for the publication of the data and images that appear in the article.

Data Availability Statement: Not applicable.

Conflicts of Interest: The authors declare that E.A. is the Scientific Director and S.P. and R.P. are scientists at BTI Biotechnology Institute, a biomedical company that investigates in the fields of regenerative medicine and PRGF-Endoret technology. The rest of the authors state that that they have no conflict of interest that are relevant to the content of this article.

Abbreviations

JT	Conjoined tendon
LBF	Long head of biceps femoris
PRGF	Plasma Rich in Growth Factors
PRP	Platelet-rich plasma
SMT	Tendon of semimembranous muscle
STT	Semitendinosus tendon

References

1. Matache, B.A.; Jazrawi, L. Surgical Management of Chronic Proximal Hamstring Tendon Tears. In *Proximal Hamstring Tears: From Endoscopic Repair to Open Reconstruction*; Youm, T., Ed.; Springer International Publishing: Cham, Switzerland, 2021.
2. Grasso, M.; O'Neill, C.; Constantinescu, D.; Moatshe, G.; Vap, A. Reconstruction of Chronic Proximal Hamstring Tear: Description of a Surgical Technique. *Arthrosc. Tech.* **2021**, *10*, e1307–e1313. [CrossRef]
3. Haskel, J.D. Surgical Treatment of Partial Proximal Hamstring Tendon Tears. In *Proximal Hamstring Tears: From Endoscopic Repair to Open Reconstruction*; Youm, T., Ed.; Springer International Publishing: Cham, Switzerland, 2021; pp. 45–55.
4. Sanchez, M.; Anitua, E.; Azofra, J.; Andia, I.; Padilla, S.; Mujika, I. Comparison of surgically repaired Achilles tendon tears using platelet-rich fibrin matrices. *Am. J. Sports Med.* **2007**, *35*, 245–251. [CrossRef]
5. Sanchez, M.; Anitua, E.; Delgado, D.; Prado, R.; Sanchez, P.; Fiz, N.; Guadilla, J.; Azofra, J.; Pompei, O.; Orive, G.; et al. Ultrasound-guided plasma rich in growth factors injections and scaffolds hasten motor nerve functional recovery in an ovine model of nerve crush injury. *J. Tissue Eng. Regen. Med.* **2017**, *11*, 1619–1629. [CrossRef]
6. Wood, D.G.; Packham, I.; Trikha, S.P.; Linklater, J. Avulsion of the proximal hamstring origin. *J. Bone Joint Surg. Am.* **2008**, *90*, 2365–2374. [CrossRef] [PubMed]
7. Anitua, E.; Prado, R.; Nurden, A.T.; Nurden, P. Characterization of Plasma Rich in Growth Factors (PRGF): Components and formulations. In *Platelet Rich Plasma in Orthopaedics and Sports Medicine*; Anitua, E., Cugat, R., Sánchez, M., Eds.; Springer International Publishing: Cham, Switzerland, 2018; pp. 29–45.
8. Ebert, J.R.; Gormack, N.; Annear, P.T. Reconstruction of chronic proximal hamstring avulsion injuries using ipsilateral distal hamstring tendons results in good clinical outcomes and patient satisfaction. *Knee Surg. Sports Traumatol. Arthrosc.* **2019**, *27*, 2958–2966. [CrossRef] [PubMed]
9. Rust, D.A.; Giveans, M.R.; Stone, R.M.; Samuelson, K.M.; Larson, C.M. Functional Outcomes and Return to Sports After Acute Repair, Chronic Repair, and Allograft Reconstruction for Proximal Hamstring Ruptures. *Am. J. Sports Med.* **2014**, *42*, 1377–1383. [CrossRef] [PubMed]
10. Moatshe, G.; Chahla, J.; Vap, A.R.; Ferrari, M.; Sanchez, G.; Mitchell, J.J.; LaPrade, R.F. Repair of Proximal Hamstring Tears: A Surgical Technique. *Arthrosc. Tech.* **2017**, *6*, e311–e317. [CrossRef] [PubMed]
11. Anitua, E.; Nurden, P.; Prado, R.; Nurden, A.T.; Padilla, S. Autologous fibrin scaffolds: When platelet- and plasma-derived biomolecules meet fibrin. *Biomaterials* **2019**, *192*, 440–460. [CrossRef] [PubMed]
12. Padilla, S.; Sanchez, M.; Vaquerizo, V.; Malanga, G.A.; Fiz, N.; Azofra, J.; Rogers, C.J.; Samitier, G.; Sampson, S.; Seijas, R.; et al. Platelet-Rich Plasma Applications for Achilles Tendon Repair: A Bridge between Biology and Surgery. *Int. J. Mol. Sci.* **2021**, *22*, 824. [CrossRef] [PubMed]
13. De Vitis, R.; Passiatore, M.; Perna, A.; Fioravanti Cinci, G.; Taccardo, G. Comparison of Shape Memory Staple and Gelled Platelet-Rich Plasma versus Shape Memory Staple alone for the Treatment of Waist Scaphoid Nonunion: A Single-Center Experience. *Joints* **2019**, *7*, 84–90. [CrossRef] [PubMed]
14. Sanchez, M.; Delgado, D.; Sanchez, P.; Fiz, N.; Azofra, J.; Orive, G.; Anitua, E.; Padilla, S. Platelet rich plasma and knee surgery. *Biomed. Res. Int.* **2014**, *2014*, 890630. [CrossRef] [PubMed]

MDPI
St. Alban-Anlage 66
4052 Basel
Switzerland
www.mdpi.com

Journal of Clinical Medicine Editorial Office
E-mail: jcm@mdpi.com
www.mdpi.com/journal/jcm

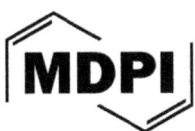

Disclaimer/Publisher's Note: The statements, opinions and data contained in all publications are solely those of the individual author(s) and contributor(s) and not of MDPI and/or the editor(s). MDPI and/or the editor(s) disclaim responsibility for any injury to people or property resulting from any ideas, methods, instructions or products referred to in the content.

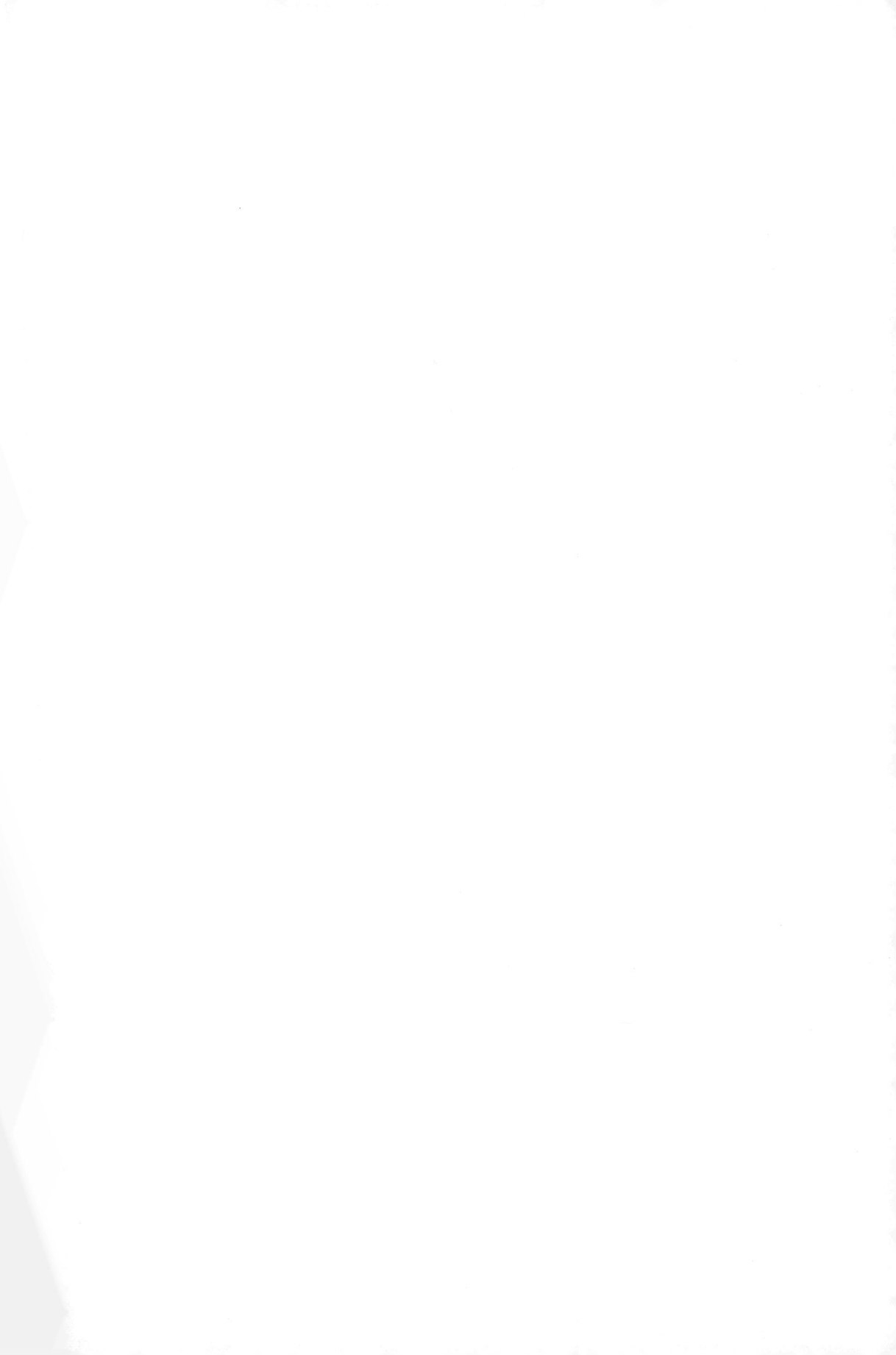

www.ingramcontent.com/pod-product-compliance
Lightning Source LLC
LaVergne TN
LVHW070601100526
838202LV00012B/536